Handbook of Psychopharmacotherapy

A Life Span Approach

Handbook of Psychopharmacotherapy

A Life Span Approach

Mani N. Pavuluri, MD, PhD, FRANZCP
Assistant Professor
Director
Pediatric Mood Disorders Clinic
and Bipolar Research Program
University of Illinois at Chicago

Philip G. Janicak, MD
Professor of Psychiatry and Pharmacology
Medical Director
Psychiatric Clinical Research Center
Rush University
Chicago, Illinois

LIPPINCOTT WILLIAMS & WILKINS
A **Wolters Kluwer** Company
Philadelphia • Baltimore • New York • London
Buenos Aires • Hong Kong • Sydney • Tokyo

Acquisitions Editor: Charles W. Mitchell
Developmental Editor: Lisa R. Kairis
Supervising Editor: Mary Ann McLaughlin
Production Editor: Barbara Stabb, TechBooks
Manufacturing Manager: Colin J. Warnock
Cover Designer: Brian Crede
Compositor: TechBooks
Printer: RR Donnelley, Crawfordsville

Library of Congress Cataloging-in-Publication Data

Pavuluri, Mani N.
  Handbook of psychopharmacotherapy : a life span approach / Mani N.
Pavuluri, Philip G. Janicak.
      p. ; cm.
  Includes bibliographical references and index.
  ISBN 0-7817-5356-2
  1. Psychopharmacology—Handbooks, manuals, etc.   2. Pediatric
psychopharmacology—Handbooks, manuals, etc.   3. Geriatric
psychopharmacology—Handbooks, manuals, etc.   I. Janicak, Philip G.
II. Title.
  [DNLM: 1. Psychotropic Drugs—pharmacology—Handbooks.   2. Age
Factors—Handbooks.   QV 39 P339h 2004]
RM315.P37   2004
615′.78—dc22

                                                            2004005868

Care has been taken to confirm the accuracy of the information presented and
to describe generally accepted practices. However, the authors and publisher
are not responsible for errors or omissions or for any consequences from
application of the information in this book and make no warranty, expressed
or implied, with respect to the currency, completeness, or accuracy of the
contents of the publication. Application of this information in a particular
situation remains the professional responsibility of the practitioner.
  The authors and publisher have exerted every effort to ensure that drug
selection and dosage set forth in this text are in accordance with current
recommendations and practice at the time of publication. However, in view of
ongoing research, changes in government regulations, and the constant flow
of information relating to drug therapy and drug reactions, the reader is
urged to check the package insert for each drug for any change in indications
and dosage and for added warnings and precautions. This is particularly
important when the recommended agent is a new or infrequently employed
drug.
  Some drugs and medical devices presented in this publication have Food
and Drug Administration (FDA) clearance for limited use in restricted
research settings. It is the responsibility of the health care provider to
ascertain the FDA status of each drug or device planned for use in their
clinical practice.

                                    10 9 8 7 6 5 4 3 2 1

Contents

Preface

This book is for all clinicians who practice psychopharmacotherapy across the life span and who need succinct and credible information to guide them in prescribing. This book is also for medical students, residents, and fellows in clinical settings involving children, adolescents, adults, and the elderly. It does not teach decision making about how to choose a drug for a specific disorder or symptom. Rather, it provides relevant information on a chosen drug. In addition, the book provides a quick reference about a drug's relative advantages and disadvantages in comparison to available alternatives. Information on drugs used to manage substance abuse, not readily available in most conventional textbooks, is also provided.

Although every attempt is made to be current, the reader must take into account that FDA-approved indications and preparations can change rapidly, with new drugs and formulations frequently being added to our current repertoire. In summary, we offer information on available formulations, how to prescribe across the life span, how to choose alternatives, and critical cautionary concerns.

For those seeking a more complete companion reference work, we would recommend *Principles and Practice of Psychopharmacotherapy,* 3rd edition (Janicak et al., 2001).

We want to thank Drs. Bhargavi Devineni, and Abid Nazeer, Ms. Katherine Kerr, and Ms. Marissa Benni for their invaluable help in the preparation of this handbook.

Mani N. Pavuluri and Philip G. Janicak

First-generation Antipsychotics

Mechanism of Action

Central dopamine receptor (e.g., D_2, D_3, and D_4) blockade. First-generation antipsychotics (FGAs) induce depolarization of dopamine neurons in nigrostriatal, mesolimbic, or other pathways (Table 1-1, Fig. 1-1).

Possible Advantage

Decreased dopaminergic activity improves certain symptoms of psychosis (e.g., positive symptoms)

Side Effects

Central Nervous System
- Extrapyramidal symptoms (EPS): major side effect of FGAs; incidence of EPS is directly proportional to the potency of FGAs.
  Acute EPS
  - Parkinsonian syndrome (occurs early in treatment and tends to persist if not treated)
  - Acute dystonia (occurs early in treatment and tends to persist if not treated)
  - Akathisia
  Late-onset (tardive) EPS: usually occurs after several months to years of drug exposure.
  - Buccolinguomasticatory movements: sucking, smacking of lips
  - Choreoathetoid movements of tongue
  - Choreiform/athetoid movements of extremities and/or truncal areas
  - Any combination of these symptoms
- Sedation: inversely proportional to milligram potency. Usually occurs within a few days of treatment initiation (due to antihistamine action). Can be avoided by shifting to a less sedating agent or giving the entire dose at bedtime.
- Neuroleptic malignant syndrome: requires early recognition, immediate discontinuation of medication, supportive measures (e.g., cooling blankets) and other treatment (e.g., dantrolene)

Anticholinergic Effects

Blurred vision, dry mouth, constipation, urinary retention; cognitive disruption

1

Table 1-1. Commonly used first-generation antipsychotics

Generic Name	Trade Name	Half-life (hr)	Dose Range (mg) per Day		Potency	Comments
			Adults	Children		
Chlorpromazine	Thorazine	24 (8–35)	100–1,000	Approved for children older than 6 mo	Low	• Sedation and ortho-static hypotension are common side effects.
			10–200	6 mo to 12 yr: • Oral—0.25 mg/kg q.i.d. or b.i.d. • Rectal—1 mg/kg q.i.d. or t.i.d. • IM—0.5 mg/kg q.i.d. or t.i.d. Adolescents: 10 mg t.i.d. to 25 mg q.i.d.		• Photosensitivity, jaundice, and ocular deposits at higher doses are specific side effects.
Haloperidol	Haldol	24 (12–36)	3–30 0.25–4	Approved for children older than 3 yr, 0.5–2 mg/d	High	• Significant EPS
Thioridazine	Mellaril	24 (6–40)	30–800 10–200	Approved for children older than 2 yr 2–12 yr: 0.5 mg/kg/d to a maximum of 3 mg/kg/d	Low	• Higher incidence of cardiac rhythm disturbances • Retinitis pigmentosa at doses >800 mg/d

					Pediatric	Potency	Comments
					Older than 12 yr: As in adults		
Mesoridazine	Serentil	30 (24–48)	20–200	10–200	No information available	Low	• Delayed ejaculation; only used for treatment resistance or intolerance • Available in parenteral form • Prolonged QT
Molindone	Moban	12 (6–24)	15–225 Elderly should be started on low dose.		Approved for children older than 12 yr, 50–70 mg/d initial dose and increased to 100 mg/d in 3–4 d	Medium	• May cause less weight gain
Fluphenazine	Prolixin	18 (14–24)	5–40	0.25–4	Approved for children older than 12 yr, 2.5–10 mg q.i.d. or t.i.d.	High	• Available in long-acting formulation
Trifluoperazine	Stelazine	18 (14–24)	2–30	1–15	Approved for children older than 6 yr 6–12 yr: 1 mg q.i.d. or b.i.d. Adolescents: 1–5 mg b.i.d.; optimal dose is 15–20 mg/d	High	—

(continued)

Table 1-1. (*Continued*)

Generic Name	Trade Name	Half-life (hr)	Dose Range (mg) per Day		Potency	Comments
			Adults	Children		
Thiothixene	Navane	34	6–40 1–15	Approved for children older than 12 yr; no specific dose for children	High	—
Perphenazine	Trilafon	12 (8–21)	2–12 2–32	No information available	High	—
Loxapine	Loxitane	8 (3–12)	20–250 10–100	Approved for children older than 16 yr; same as adults	Medium	—
Pimozide	Orap	55 (29–111)	1–10 0.25–4	Approved for children older than 12 yr, 0.2 mg/kg/d; maximum, 10 mg/d	High	—

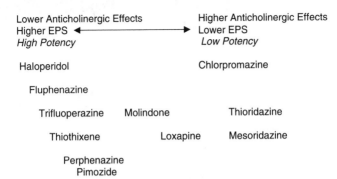

FIG. 1-1. **First-generation antipsychotic side effects.**

Cardiovascular System
- Alpha-adrenergic blockade: orthostatic hypotension; reflex tachycardia
- Cardiac rhythm disturbances: prolongation of QT interval, torsade de pointes (especially thioridazine)

Endocrine Effects
- Decreased dopamine activity in the pituitary increases prolactin levels
- May cause breast engorgement and lactation in women and gynecomastia in men, as well as sexual dysfunction in both genders

Weight Gain
Less compared with some second-generation antipsychotics

Drug Interactions
Avoid concomitant use with antacids, barbiturates, and lithium, which may decrease efficacy or increase toxicity.

Second-generation Antipsychotics

CLOZAPINE

Chemical Group
Dibenzodiazepine

Trade Name
Clozaril (Novartis Pharmaceuticals)

Forms Available
Caplets of 25 and 100 mg

Pharmacokinetics
Half-life is 5 to 15 hours, peaks in 1 to 4 hours, steady state in 3 to 4 days, bioavailability 60%.

Dispensing
12.5 to 25 mg per day, then 25 mg b.i.d., increasing by 25 mg per day after reaching 100 mg. Dose is increased over a month. Wait long enough to assess for effects without increasing the dose. Taper carefully as cholinergic rebound/psychosis or other withdrawal symptoms may occur, including nausea, vomiting, diarrhea, and increased salivation.

Range of Dosing
Adults: 25 to 900 mg per day.
Children: start at 12.5 mg once per day and gradually increase to no more than 3 to 6 mg per kg per day in divided doses.
Elderly: 10 to 100 mg per day. May be too sedating and respiratory problems have been reported in the elderly.

FDA Approval
Treatment-resistant schizophrenia; suicidal behavior in schizophrenia and schizoaffective disorder.

Possible Mechanism of Action
Higher ratio of serotonin to dopamine antagonism: D_{1++}, D_2, D_3, D_{4+}, $5HT_{2c\ 2a++}$

Possible Advantages
- Treatment-resistant psychosis, including schizophrenia, schizoaffective disorder, bipolar disorder
- May decrease suicidality in schizophrenia and schizoaffective disorder (only agent with this Food and Drug Administration (FDA) indication)
- Patients may continue to improve for 12 months or longer
- EPS does not usually occur across recommended dosing range; substantial decrease in tardive dyskinesia
- May improve negative symptoms (directly or indirectly)

Side Effects
- Agranulocytosis (see following section)
- Anticholinergic side effects
- Hypersalivation, especially nocturnal
- Tachycardia, low-grade fever, shorter QTc interval (due to vagal inhibition)
- Weight gain: H_1 and $5HT_{2c}$ antagonism
- Seizures (1% to 2%): increased risk (3% to 5%) if dose is greater than or equal to 600 mg per day; may need to use anticonvulsant concomitantly, avoid carbamazepine
- Postural hypotension: α_1 antagonism
- Sedation: H_1 and α_1 antagonism (tolerance develops based on dose)
- Nocturnal enuresis
- Neuroleptic malignant syndrome
- Dyslipidemia
- Myocarditis
- New-onset diabetes; diabetic ketoacidosis (DKA)

Agranulocytosis
Decrease in number of polymorphonuclear leukocytes (PMNL) (i.e., absolute neutrophil count) less than 0.5% compared with 1% to 2%
   Idiosyncratic reaction, not dose related

Drug Interactions
Cimetidine, erythromycin, selective serotonin reuptake inhibitors (SSRIs), caffeine intake, smoking cessation, or risperidone may increase clozapine level

Risk
Risk is less than 0.5% and other factors include:

- 95% of the cases in first 6 months
- Highest in first 4 to 18 weeks
- Women greater than men
- Older age
- Ethnicity

- If increased/decreased white blood (cell) count (WBC), increased erythrocyte sedimentation rate (ESR)

Management[1]
- 3,500 (or has dropped by a substantial amount from baseline): counts should be repeated
- 3,500 and/or the granulocyte count falls below 1,500: monitor twice weekly with differentials
- 3,000 and/or granulocyte count less than 1,500: interrupt treatment and obtain CBC and differentials daily. May resume if no symptoms of infection and WBC returns to more than 3,000 plus more than 1,500 granulocyte count. Continue twice weekly monitoring until WBC is more than 3,500
- 2,000 or granulocytes less than 1,000: stop clozapine and place the patient in reverse isolation with daily CBC and differential until levels return to normal. Do not rechallenge with clozapine

Tests
For agranulocytosis, initially, draw complete blood cell count (CBC) and differential count weekly; after 6 months, biweekly.

Plasma levels: 350 to 450 ng per mL for parent compound.

[1] From Janicak PG, Davis JM, Perskorn SH, Ayd, FA. *Principles and Practice of Psychopharmacotherapy*, 3rd ed. Philadelphia: Lippincott Williams & Wilkins, 2001.

RISPERIDONE

Chemical Group
Benzisoxazole

Trade Name
Risperdal (Janssen Pharmaceutica)
Risperdal Consta (IM form) (Janssen-Cilag)

Forms Available
Tablets of 0.25, 0.5, 1, 2, 3, and 4 mg; elixir 1 mg per mL in 100-mg bottle; m-TAB rapid dissolve formulation 0.5 mg, 1 mg, 2 mg; risperidone Consta (microspheres) 25 mg, 37.5, 50 mg IM.

Pharmacokinetics
Half-life is 3 hours in fast metabolizers and 20 hours in poor metabolizers; half-life of its major metabolite 9-OH-risperidone is 21 to 30 hours; peaks in 1 to 3 hours; steady state in 1 to 5 days; bioavailability 70%.

Dispensing
Once a day is effective, but usually start as b.i.d. dose in adults and may continue as b.i.d. in children.

Range of Dosing
Adults: usual range is 2 to 6 mg per day. Risperidone Consta is usually given for adults 25 mg IM once every 2 weeks. Oral dose of 2–3 mg is given for the first 3 weeks. Maximum recommended dose is 50 mg IM.
Children: start at 0.25 once or twice a day and gradually increase to 4 mg. Weight-based calculation is 0.1 to 0.5 mg per kg per day.
Elderly: 0.25 to 2 mg per day. May be activating, can cause EPS.

FDA Approval
Manifestations of psychotic disorders; bipolar mania and mixed episodes

Possible Mechanism of Action
Serotonin-dopamine antagonism: $5HT_{2a}$ is greater than D_2, preferentially distributed in frontal cortex and striatum. D_2 antagonism reduces dopamine in prefrontal cortex; may improve positive symptoms; $5HT_2$ antagonism may improve negative and mood symptoms. No appreciable affinity for muscarinic cholinergic receptors.

Possible Advantages
- Improve positive symptoms
- Improve mood symptoms
- May decrease negative symptoms
- May decrease cognitive symptoms
- Less anticholinergic side effects
- Long-acting formulation

Side Effects
- Increased risk of extrapyramidal symptoms, especially with dosages above 6 mg per day
- Postural hypotension: α_1 antagonism
- Increased prolactin: D_2 antagonism
- Weight gain, sedation, decreased concentration
- 9-OH metabolite: QTc interval increased, clinical significance unknown
- Dyslipidemia
- New-onset diabetes; DKA

Pregnancy
Discontinue gradually 2 weeks before due date to avoid extrapyramidal symptoms in newborns. It is present in breast milk.

Drug Interactions
Metabolized by CYP 2D6; therefore, potentially subject to interactions with inhibitors such as fluoxetine, which may increase risperidone level.

Tests
Check prolactin levels, if symptomatic.

OLANZAPINE

Chemical Group
Thienobenzodiazepine

Trade Name
Zyprexa (Eli Lilly)

Forms Available
Tablets of 2.5, 5, 7.5, 10, 15, and 20 mg; Zydis rapid dissolve formulation, contains phenylalanine; acute parenteral formulation (not yet available).

Pharmacokinetics
Half-life is 31 hours, peaks in 6 hours; steady state in 7 days; bioavailability 60%.

Dispensing
Once a day dosing

Range of Dosing
Adults: usually 5 to 20 mg per day. Although the recommended maximum dose is 20 mg, this is often exceeded.
Children: 0.12 to 0.20 mg/kg body weight, given in 1 to 3 divided doses.
Elderly: 2.5 to 10 mg per day.

FDA Approval
Schizophrenia, bipolar mania, bipolar depression (combined with fluoxetine; see symbyax, Appendix F, for more details)

Possible Mechanism of Action
Serotonin-dopamine antagonist: $5HT_2$; D_1, D_2, D_3, D_4

Possible Advantages
- Decrease positive symptoms
- Improve mood symptoms
- May decrease negative symptoms
- May improve cognitive symptoms
- No significant electrocardiogram (ECG) changes

Side Effects
- D_2: increased prolactin (temporary, not sustained); akathisia may be seen with higher doses
- α_1: orthostatic hypotension, dizziness, and syncope
- M_1 to M_5: anticholinergic side effects
- H_1;$5HT_{2C}$: weight gain; somnolence
- New-onset diabetes; DKA

Drug Interactions
- Benzodiazepines: orthostatic hypotension, syncope
- Carbamazepine, rifampin: lower olanzapine level
- Cimetidine, fluvoxamine, smoking cessation: increase olanzapine level

Tests
- Hepatic: increased serum glutamate pyruvate transferase (SGPT)
- Dyslipidemia
- Glucose levels

QUETIAPINE

Chemical Group
Dibenzothiazepine

Trade Name
Seroquel (AstraZeneca)

Forms Available
Tablets of 25, 100, 200, and 300 mg. Sustained release tablets and granule sachets are currently being studied.

Pharmacokinetics
Half-life is 7 hours, peak in 1.5 hours; steady state in 2 days.

Dispensing
B.i.d. dosing

Range of Dosing
Adults: 75 to 750 mg per day. Although the recommended maximum dose is 800 mg, this is often exceeded.
Children: start at 12.5 mg or 25 mg once or twice a day and gradually increase to a maximum of 3 to 6 mg per kg per day in divided doses.
Elderly: 25 to 300 mg per day.

FDA Approval
Manifestations of psychotic disorders; bipolar mania

Possible Mechanism of Action
Serotonin-dopamine antagonism: $5HT_{2+++}$, $5HT_{6++}$, D_{1+}, D_{2+}, D_4. No appreciable affinity for muscarinic cholinergic receptors.

Possible Advantages
- Decrease positive symptoms
- Improve mood symptoms
- May decrease negative symptoms
- May improve cognitive symptoms
- Extrapyramidal side effects are negligible across entire dosing range
- Nonsustained prolactin elevation across entire dosing range
- No significant ECG changes

Side Effects
- α_1: orthostatic hypotension, dizziness, syncope
- H_1: risk of somnolence higher during the 3 to 5 days of initial dose titration
- Transient increase in weight and hepatic enzymes, and decreases in total and free T_4
- Dyslipidemia
- New-onset diabetes; DKA

Drug Interactions
Metabolized by CYP 3A4, therefore potentially subject to interactions with ketoconazole and erythromycin, increasing quetiapine level. Thioridazine, phenytoin, and carbamazepine can decrease quetiapine level.

Tests
Prescribing information recommends slit lamp eye exam at baseline and every 6 months with long-term treatment for those at risk to develop cataracts. A causal relationship between cataract formation and quetiapine in humans has not been established.

ZIPRASIDONE

Chemical Group
Benzisothiazol

Trade Name
Geodon (Pfizer, Inc.)

Forms Available
Capsules of 20, 40, 60, and 80 mg. Injection of single-dose vial, 20 mg per mL, for acute parenteral use only.

Pharmacokinetics
Half-life is 7 hours, peaks in 6 to 8 hours; steady state in 2 to 3 days; bioavailability increased two-fold with food to 60%.

Dispensing
B.i.d. dosing

Range of Dosing
Adults: efficacy was observed in dose range of 20 to 80 mg b.i.d. Maximum recommended dose is 160 mg. Dose is raised after a minimum of 2 days.
Children: start at 20 mg b.i.d. and gradually increase to no more than 40 mg b.i.d. Comes in capsules and cannot be administered at lower doses to preschool-age population. The optimal dosage in children has not been determined.
Elderly: There is no indication for reduced clearance of ziprasidone; however, due to multiple factors that may increase pharmacodynamic response or cause poorer tolerance or orthostasis, a lower starting dose and careful monitoring during the initial period should be considered.

FDA Approval
Psychotic disorders

Possible Mechanism of Action
Serotonin-dopamine antagonism: $5HT_{2a}$, $5HT_{1d}$, D_2 and D_3 antagonist, and $5HT_{1a}$ partial agonist. It is also an SSRI and a norepinephrine reuptake inhibitor. No appreciable affinity for muscarinic cholinergic receptors.

Possible Advantages
• Decrease positive symptoms
• Improve mood symptoms

- May decrease negative symptoms
- May improve cognitive symptoms
- No prolactin elevation, no substantial weight gain
- Minimal risk of extrapyramidal symptoms

Side Effects
- Dose-related QTc prolongation (Fig. 2-1).
- Contraindicated in patients with known history of QT prolongation:
  - Congenital long QT syndrome
  - Recent acute myocardial infarction (MI) or uncompensated heart failure

  Risk is increased in patients with:
  - Bradycardia
  - Hypokalemia/hypomagnesemia
  - Concurrent drugs causing QT prolongation
- α_1 antagonism: postural hypotension, especially during initial dosing period
- Upper respiratory symptoms, sedation
- Pregnancy: discontinue gradually 2 weeks before due date to avoid extrapyramidal symptoms in newborns. Present in breast milk.
- New-onset diabetes; DKA

Tests

Prescribing information recommends baseline K^+ and Mg^{++} measurements. Baseline ECG in children (not an FDA requirement, but suggested in patients with potassium or sodium imbalance).

ARIPIPRAZOLE

Chemical Group
Quinolinone

Trade Name
Abilify (Bristol-Myers and Otsuka America Pharmaceuticals)

Forms Available
Tablets 5, 10, 15, 20, and 30 mg

Pharmacokinetics
Half-life is 75 hours; half-life of its major metabolite, dehydroaripiprazole is 94 hours, peaks in 3 to 5 hours; steady state in 14 days; bioavailability 87%.

Dispensing
Once a day, with or without food. However, due to possible nausea, administration with a meal is advised.

Range of Dosing
Adults: recommended starting and target dose is 15 mg per day. Dose increase should be made after 2 to 3 weeks because this timeframe is needed to achieve steady state.
Children: no information is available yet. Due to side effects such as nausea, it is recommended that aripiprazole be started at a lower dose (2.5 to 5 mg) and gradually increased.
Elderly: lower starting dose is recommended because safety and efficacy have not been established in patients with psychosis associated with dementia.

FDA Approval
Schizophrenia, bipolar mania (pending)

Possible Mechanism of Action
Partial agonist at D_2 and $5HT_{1A}$ receptors and antagonist at postsynaptic $5HT_{2A}$ receptors. Partial agonist activity at D_2 and $5HT_{1A}$ is hypothesized to stabilize these neurotransmitter systems.

Aripiprazole exhibits
High affinity for D_2 (partial agonist), D_3, $5HT_{1A}$ (partial agonist), and $5HT_{2A}$ receptors

Moderate affinity for D_4, $5HT_{2c}$, $5HT_7$, α_1, and H_1 receptors and serotonin reuptake site

No appreciable affinity for muscarinic cholinergic receptors

Possible Advantages
- Decrease positive symptoms
- Improve mood symptoms
- May decrease negative symptoms
- May improve cognitive symptoms
- Minimal EPS
- No prolactin increase
- Minimal weight gain
- No clinically significant changes in hematological, serum chemistry, and urinalysis parameters
- No significant ECG changes

Side Effects
- Most common: headache (32%), nausea (14%), vomiting (12%), constipation (10%), anxiety (25%), insomnia (24%), dizziness (11%), akathisia (10%). EPS all types 6%, similar to placebo.
- Dose-related side effect: somnolence
- Weight gain: study data looks favorable
- New-onset diabetes; DKA (study data looks favorable)

Pregnancy
Caution: Safety in pregnancy is not established. Not recommended during breast feeding.

Metabolism and Drug Interaction
Aripiprazole is metabolized by biotransformation pathways: dehydrogenation (CYP 3A4 and CYP 2D6), hydroxylation, and N-dealkylation (CYP 3A4) by P450 enzymes.

Agents that induce CYP 3A4 (e.g., phenytoin, carbamazepine, rifampin) could cause increases in aripiprazole clearance, resulting in the need for higher doses. Inhibitors of CYP 3A4 (e.g., ketoconazole, fluoxetine, fluvoxamine) and CYP 2D6 (e.g., fluoxetine, paroxetine, quinidine) can inhibit aripiprazole elimination and cause increased blood levels. Dose should be adjusted accordingly.

Maximum   **Minimum**

ACUTE EPS

←···→

Haloperidol   Risperidone   Olanzapine   Clozapine
                                                       Ziprasidone
                           (Dose related)   Quetiapine
                                                       Aripiprazole

PROLACTIN ELEVATION

←···→

Haloperidol   Ziprasidone   Clozapine
Risperidone   Quetiapine
                                   Olanzapine   Aripiprazole

QTc INTERVAL

←···→

Thioridazine   Ziprasidone   Risperidone
Mesoridazine   Olanzapine
                           Quetiapine Haloperidol
                                      Aripiprazole

WEIGHT GAIN

←···→

Clozapine   Quetiapine   Ziprasidone
    Olanzapine   Risperidone   Haloperidol
                                                  Aripiprazole

FIG. 2-1.   Dose-related QTc prolongation. (Adapted from Jan-icak PG, Davis JM, Perskorn SH, Ayd, FJ. *Principles and Practice of Psychopharmacotherapy,* 3rd ed. Philadelphia: Lippincott Williams & Wilkins, 2001.)

First-generation Antidepressants

Chemical Group
Heterocyclics (HCAs)
Monoamine oxidase inhibitors (MAOIs)

Trade Name
Refer to Table 3-1 for trade names.

Forms Available
- HCAs: tablets, capsules, and concentrate (see Table 3-1 for dose ranges)
- MAOIs: tablets
  - Phenelzine 15 mg
  - Tranylcypromine 10 mg

Pharmacokinetics

HCAs

- Half-lives are usually 24 to 30 hours
- Therapeutic plasma levels include:

  Notriptyline: 50 to 170 ng per mL
  Desimpramine: 110 to 160 ng per mL
  Amitriptyline: 80 to 150 ng per mL
  Imipramine: ~250 ng per mL (threshold)

- Significant first-pass metabolism
- Substrates for CYP 2D6, CYP 3A3/4
- Highly protein bound
- Highly lipophilic

MAOIs

- Half-lives are short (i.e., 2 to 4 hours), but half-life of MAO inhibition is about 2 weeks because it takes that period to synthesize the new enzyme
- Undergo "first-pass" degradation, so alterations in metabolism (genetic, acquired) could affect bioavailability and/or efficacy

Dispensing
Initially, twice daily until optimal dose is determined and acclimation to side effects is achieved. Then usually can administer once daily. If higher doses (e.g., 250 to 300 mg per day) are required, may need to give b.i.d. to minimize side effects.

Table 3-1.   First-generation antidepressants

Drug	Trade Name	Dose Range (mg/d)
Heterocyclics		
Amitriptyline	Elavil	75–300
Imipramine	Tofranil	75–300
Doxepin	Sinequan	75–300
Desipramine	Norpramin	75–300
Nortriptyline	Pamelor	75–300
Trimipramine	Surmontil	75–200
Protriptyline	Vivactil	20–60
Clomipramine	Anafranil	100–250
Maprotiline	Ludiomil	75–225
Dibenzoxazepine		
Amoxapine	Ascendin	200–600
Phenylpiperazine		
Trazodone	Desyrel	150–600
Monoamine oxidase inhibitors		
Phenelzine	Nardil	15–90
Tranylcypromine	Parnate	30–60

Range of Dosing

Refer to Table 3-1 for dose ranges.

FDA Approval

HCAs: depression, obsessive-compulsive disorder (OCD) (clomipramine)

MAOIs: depression; atypical depression

Possible Mechanism of Action

- Norepinephrine (NE) and serotonin (5HT) reuptake inhibition
- Monoamine oxidase (A, B)
  - Nonselective (A **and** B) or selective (A **or** B)
  - Irreversible or reversible
- HCAs
  - Downregulation of NE and 5HT receptors
- MAOIs
  - Irreversible inhibition of MAO by covalently bonding to the enzyme (e.g., phenelzine, tranylcypromine)
  - Newer agents may be selective for MAO-A (e.g., clorgyline) or MAO-B (e.g., l-deprenyl) and reversibly inhibit the enzyme (e.g., moclobemide)

Table 3-2. Side effects of first-generation antidepressants

Drugs	Sedation	Anticholinergic	Orthostatic Hypotension	Cardiac Effects
Heterocyclics				
Amitriptyline	High	High	Moderate	High
Clomipramine	High	High	Low	Moderate
Desipramine	Low	Low	Low	Moderate
Doxepin	High	Moderate	Moderate	Moderate
Imipramine	Moderate	Moderate	High	High
Maprotiline	Moderate	Moderate	Low	Moderate
Nortriptyline	Moderate	Moderate	Low	Moderate
Protriptyline	Low	Moderate	Low	Moderate
Trimipramine	High	High	Moderate	High
Dibenzoxazapines				
Amoxapine[a]	Low	Low	None	None
Phenylpiperazine				
Trazodone	High	Low	Moderate	Low
Monoamine oxidase inhibitors				
Phenelzine	Low	None	High	None
Tranylcypromine	High	Very low	Very low	None

[a]May cause EPS due to active metabolite effects.

Anatomic sites of action
- Locus coeruleus
- Raphe nuclei

Possible Advantages

HCAs may be more effective for severe depression, whereas MAOIs may be more effective for atypical depression.

Side Effects

For adverse effects, refer to Table 3-2; cardiac arrhythmias most serious and potentially lethal.

Drug Interactions

HCAs
- CYP 2D6 substrates, so metabolism will be altered by inhibitors or inducers of this isoenzyme

MAOIs
- May cause life-threatening serotonin syndrome when combined with other potent serotonin agents (e.g., SSRIs)

Second-generation Antidepressants

FLUOXETINE

Chemical Group
(+/−)-N-methyl-3-phenyl-3-[α,α,α-trifluoro-p-tolyl)-oxy] propylamine hydrochloride

Trade Name
Prozac (Eli Lilly)

Forms Available
Capsules of 10, 20, and 40 mg; elixir 20 mg per 5 mL (mint flavored); long-acting form (Prozac Weekly) available as 90-mg capsule, with a booster pack of four tablets for a month's supply.

Pharmacokinetics
Half-life is 1 to 3 days for fluoxetine (increases to 4 to 6 days with chronic administration); 7 to 9 days for norfluoxetine. Prozac Weekly is the delayed-release form given once a week. It consists of enteric-coated pellets released in the small bowel. Peak concentration in blood is same as the 20-mg tablet, but troughs and steady-state concentrations are lower than the immediate-release (IR) tablets given once daily. Plasma concentrations may not be predictive of clinical response.

Dispensing
Once a day. Long-acting form starts to release medication in 10 hours. When making the transition from IR to long-acting form relation, need a week's overlap with both medications. Separate the first 90-mg weekly dose and the last 20-mg once daily dose by one week.

FDA Approval
Depression, OCD, bulimia nervosa, panic disorder, premenstrual dysphoric disorder (PMDD)

Possible Mechanism of Action
Inhibition of 5-HT reuptake transport mechanism

Range of Dosing
Adults: starting dose is 20 mg in adults; maximum of 80 mg per day. Wait 4 weeks to increase the dose.

Children: start at 5 to 10 mg if anxious (20 mg if they are teenagers) once a day and gradually increase it to a maximum of 0.25 to 1 mg per kg per day.

Elderly: 5 to 40 mg per day. An upper dose range has not been established for the elderly; may be activating and cause insomnia; long half-life.

OCD: higher maintenance dose, response in 12 to 26 weeks.

Panic Disorder: starting dose must be very low, maintenance dose is higher. Target symptoms may first worsen; usually more than 50% improvement in symptoms is eventually observed.

Bulimia: higher starting dose, higher maintenance dose; effect in 3 to 8 weeks.

Site of Action
Serotonin reuptake transporter

Possible Mechanism of Action
- Pre- and postsynaptic receptors are upregulated secondary to depletion of 5HT
- With SSRI, 5HT is increased in somatodendritic area, then downregulates $5HT_{1A}$ autoreceptors
- More 5HT is released
- Downregulation of serotonin post- and presynaptic receptors then occurs

Anatomical Sites of Action in Central Nervous System and Indications/Actions
- Midbrain raphe–frontal lobe: depression
- Basal ganglia: OCD
- Hippocampus: panic disorder
- Hypothalamus: bulimia
- Spinal cord: pain

Possible Advantages
No adverse cardiovascular effects, wide therapeutic index

Side Effects
- $5HT_2$: agitation, akathisia, anxiety, panic, insomnia; subsides over time
- $5HT_3$: diarrhea, gastrointestinal (GI) distress and nausea (particularly high with 'Prozac Weekly')
- Central nervous system (CNS): headache
- Sexual dysfunction: due to dopamine lowering and 5HT increase in mesolimbic area and at the level of autonomic nervous system; possibly mediated by $5HT_2$; lower dose or switch to mirtazapine, bupropion or nefazodone

- Possible long-term side effects: apathy; sexual dysfunction (do not increase the dose if secondary to depression).

Drug Interactions
- Inhibits CYP 2D6—may elevate plasma levels of pimozide, phenytoin, carbamazepine, desipramine, imipramine, amitriptyline, nortriptyline, and certain antiarrhythmics.
- Stop at least 5 weeks before starting an MAOI or thioridazine.

SERTRALINE

Chemical Group
(1S-cis)-4-(3,4-dichlorophenyl)-1,2,3,4-tetrahydro-N-methyl-1-nanphthalenamine hydrochloride

Trade Name
Zoloft (Pfizer)

Forms Available
Tablets of 25, 50, and 100 mg; syrup also available, but tastes bad.

Pharmacokinetics
Half-life is 25 hours, metabolites 60 to 70 hours allowing for easier withdrawal.

Dispensing
Once a day

Range of Dosing
Adults: 25 to 200 mg per day.
Children: start at 25 mg once a day and gradually increase to no more than 100 mg for 4 to 6 weeks, then increase the dose further if necessary and if tolerated. Usually, give no more than 1.5 to 3 mg per kg per day.
Elderly: 12.5 to 150 mg per day. Can cause nausea and GI upset; may be sedating.

FDA Approval
Depression, OCD (adults and children), posttraumatic stress disorder (PTSD), panic disorder, and premenstrual dysphoric disorder (PMDD)

Possible Mechanism of Action
Inhibition of 5-HT reuptake transport mechanism

Possible Advantages
- Once a day dosing
- Fewer withdrawal symptoms
- Possibly less activating than fluoxetine
- Fewer anticholinergic side effects

Side Effects
- As in all SSRIs
- $5HT_3$ greater than in the periphery: more diarrhea compared with others
- Can cause agitation, akathisia

Drug Interactions
- Inhibits CYP 2D6: contraindicated for use with pimozide due to potential elevation of pimozide levels; may also increase levels of desipramine, imipramine, amitriptyline, nortriptyline, and certain antiarrhythmics.
- Stop at least 2 weeks before starting an MAOI or thioridazine.

PAROXETINE

Chemical Group
Phenylpiperidine-salt

Trade Name
Paxil (Smith Kline, Beecham)

Forms Available
- Tablets of 10, 20, 30, and 40 mg
- Controlled-release (CR) tablets (Paxil CR): 12.5, 25, and 37.5 mg
- Orange-flavored suspension: 10 mg per 5 mL in 250-mL bottles

Pharmacokinetics
Half-life is 24 hours for IR form and 15 to 20 hours for CR form. No active metabolites; therefore, poses a greater risk for withdrawal symptoms.

Dispensing
Once a day. CR form has a degradable polymeric matrix designed to control dissolution rate of paroxetine over a period of approximately 4 to 5 hours. Also, an enteric-coated CR form that delays start of release until tablet exits the stomach.

Range of Dosing

IR form
Adults: 10 to 60 mg per day
Children: start at 10 to 20 mg once a day. Do not exceed 0.25 to 0.70 mg per kg per day.
Elderly: 5 to 40 mg per day.

CR form
Adults: recommended initial dose is 2 mg (CR) per day for major depressive disorder and 12.5 mg for panic disorder. If not responding, increase dose in 12.5-mg increments at intervals of at least 1 week. Maximum dose not to exceed 62.5 mg for major depressive disorder and 75 mg for panic disorder.
Children: no information available yet.
Elderly: recommended initial dose is 12.5 mg per day, may be increased if necessary, not to exceed 50 mg per day.

FDA Approval
IR form: major depression, obsessive compulsive disorder (OCD), panic disorder, social anxiety disorder, general

anxiety disorder (GAD), post-traumatic stress disorder (PTSD)

CR form: major depression, panic disorder

Possible Mechanism of Action

Inhibition of 5-HT reuptake transport mechanism

Possible Advantages

Anxiety mixed with depression

Side Effects

- As in all SSRIs
- Mild anticholinergic effects
- Not good for patients with sleep difficulties

Drug Interactions

- Potent inhibitor of CYP 2D6; therefore, may increase levels of pimozide, desipramine, imipramine, amitriptyline, nortriptyline, and certain antiarrhythmics. May also inhibit its own metabolism
- Also metabolized by CYP 2D6; therefore, levels may be increased by cimetidine and decreased by phenobarbital and phenytoin.
- In case of serious hepatic and renal problems, use lower doses with maximum dose not more than 50 mg per day.
- Requires at least a 2-week washout before starting an MAOI or thioridazine.

FLUVOXAMINE

Chemical Group
2-aminoethyl oxime ether of aralkylketone

Trade Name
Luvox (Solvay Pharmaceutical)

Forms Available
Tablets of 25, 50, and 100 mg

Pharmacokinetics
Half-life 15 hours; steady state in 1 week; bioavailability is 50% and unaffected by food.

Dispensing
B.i.d.

Range of Dosing
Adults: 150 to 300 mg per day
Children: start at 25 mg b.i.d. or 50 mg once a day and increase to a tolerable and effective dose, given b.i.d. Do not exceed 1.5 to 4.5 mg per kg per day or 200 mg per day in children.
Elderly: 50 to 150 mg per day.

FDA Approval
OCD

Possible Mechanism of Action
Inhibition of 5-HT reuptake transport mechanism

Possible Advantages
Anxiety mixed with depression

Side Effects
- As in all SSRIs
- Nausea and vomiting may be higher than with other SSRIs

Drug Interactions
- Inhibits CYP 1A2; therefore, may increase levels of theophylline (decrease dose), warfarin, and propranolol.
- Inhibits CYP 3A4; therefore, contraindicated with pimozide and may increase levels of alprazolam and diazepam.
- Requires at least a 2-week washout before starting an MAOI or thioridazine.

CITALOPRAM

Chemical Group
Phthalane derivative

Trade Name
Celexa (Forest Pharmaceuticals)

Forms Available
Tablets of 10, 20, and 40 mg; peppermint solution 10 mg per 5 mL.

Pharmacokinetics
Half-life is 35 hours; steady state in 1 week; bioavailability is 80% and unaffected by food.

Dispensing
Once a day

Range of Dosing
Adults: 10 to 60 mg per day.
Children: start at 10 to 20 mg once a day. Do not exceed 0.25 to 0.70 mg per kg per day.
Elderly: recommended dose is 20 mg per day.

FDA Approval
Depression

Possible Mechanism of Action
Inhibition of 5-HT reuptake transport mechanism

Possible Advantages
Most selective SSRI; often preferred if there are multiple medical problems due to minimal drug interactions involving the CYP 450 enzyme system.

Side Effects
• As in all SSRIs
• Possibly less sexual side effects

Drug Interactions
• Weak inhibitor of CYP 2D6.
• Requires at least a 2-week washout before starting an MAOI or thioridazine.

ESCITALOPRAM

Chemical Group
Phthalane derivative, S-enantiomer of citalopram (S-CT)

Trade Name
Lexapro (Forest Pharmaceuticals)

Forms Available
Tablets of 5, 10, and 20 mg

Pharmacokinetics
Half-life 27 to 30 hours; steady state in 1 week; bioavailability is 80% and unaffected by food.

Dispensing
Once a day, with or without food (pending study); 10 and 20 mg of escitalopram is bioequivalent to 20 and 40 mg of citalopram, respectively.

Range of Dosing
Adults: 10 mg is the recommended starting and maintenance dose.
Children: no specific guidelines available yet.
Elderly: 10 mg per day for most elderly patients. However, escitalopram should be used with caution in elderly patients with decreased hepatic, renal, or cardiac function, coexistence of other diseases, as well as concomitant drug therapy.

FDA Approval
Major depressive disorder

Possible Mechanism of Action
Highly potent blockade of serotonin reuptake transport mechanism S-CT without its inactive R-enantiomer.

Possible Advantages
- No significant reuptake inhibition of norepinephrine or dopamine.
- Low affinity for serotonin, adrenergic, histamine, muscarinic, and benzodiazepine receptors.
- Minimal drug interactions involving the CYP 450 enzyme system
- Reported faster onset of action and greater overall magnitude of effect than citalopram.

Side Effects

Same as with citalopram: nausea, diarrhea, insomnia, dry mouth; possibly less sexual side effects

Drug Interactions

S-didesmethyl-CT, a metabolite of S-CT is a moderate inhibitor of CYP 2C9 and 2C19. Contraindicated with MAOIs. Needs caution when used with antimigraine medications.

VENLAFAXINE

Chemical Group
Phenethylamine bicyclic derivative

Trade Name
Effexor (Wyeth Ayerst)

Forms Available
Tablets of 25, 37.5, 50, 75, and 100 mg; extended release (XR) in 37.5-, 75-, and 150-mg capsules.

Pharmacokinetics
Half-life 5 hours; metabolite, 11 hours; steady state in 3 days.

Dispensing
Twice a day; XR available for once a day use. Withdrawal symptoms are seen with sudden cessation (e.g., gastrointestinal effects, dizziness, sweating).

Range of Dosing
Adults: 75 to 225 mg in XR form, up to 375 mg in regular form.
Children: start at 25 to 37.5 mg b.i.d. Do not exceed 1 to 3 mg per kg per day.
Elderly: No dose adjustment is recommended. As with any drug for the treatment of depression or GAD, however, caution should be used when treating the elderly, especially when increasing the dose.

FDA Approval
Depression; GAD

Possible Mechanism of Action
Serotonin and norepinephrine reuptake inhibitor (SNRI); ± Dopamine reuptake inhibitor (DRI)

Low dose: Primarily SRI (one: serotonin)
Medium dose: SRI + norepinephrine reuptake inhibitor (NRI) (two: serotonin, noradrenaline)
High dose: serotonin and norepinephrine reuptake inhibitor (SNRI) + dopamine and adrenergic reuptake inhibitor (DARI) (three: serotonin, noradrenaline, dopamine)

Possible Advantages
• Depression refractory to other agents; melancholia
• Decreased problems with weight gain, hypersomnia; may benefit atypical depression

- Reported more rapid onset of action with higher initial dose, if tolerated
- No A_1, H_1, or M_1 side effects

Side Effects
- Treatment emergent anxiety
- At higher doses, may increase blood pressure; use in hypertensive and anxious patients should be more carefully monitored
- Headache
- Insomnia
- Sweating
- Weight loss in first 5 months and then possible weight gain

Metabolism and Drug Interactions
- CYP 2D6 inhibitor
- 14-day washout prior to an MAOI or thioridazine

NEFAZODONE

Chemical Group
Phenylpiperazine

Trade Name
Serzone (Bristol-Myers Squibb)

Forms Available
Tablets of 50, 100, 150, 200, and 250 mg

Pharmacokinetics
Half-life is 2 to 4 hours; longer in elderly.

Dispensing
B.i.d. in adults; once a day is adequate in the elderly.

Range of Dosing
Adults: 200 to 600 mg; usually greater than or equal to 300 mg per day is most efficacious
Children: 1 to 8 mg per kg per day.
Elderly: 50 to 200 mg per day; upper dose range not established.

FDA Approval
Depression, generalized anxiety disorder

Possible Mechanism of Action
$5HT_2$ antagonist + serotonin reuptake inhibition (SARI, serotonin receptor antagonist and reuptake inhibitor)

Possible Advantages
Due to $5HT_2$ receptor antagonism:

- Decreased anxiety
- Increased slow-wave sleep
- Decreased sexual dysfunction

Side Effects
- A_1 antagonism-counteracted NRI = no orthostatic hypotension.
- Sedation
- Hepatotoxicity (possibly severe)

Metabolism and Drug Interactions
- CYP 3A4; metabolite formed (MCPP/$5HT_{2AC}$ agonist)
- Four percent of whites have no 2D6 to inhibit MCPP; so stimulate with opposite effect on $5HT_{2AC}$. Diagnosis

suspected if there are flulike symptoms at onset. Palinopsia secondary to partial agonism of $5HT_2$.

- Contraindicated with pimozide and carbamazepine.
- Inhibitor of CYP 3A4; therefore, may increase levels of triazolam, alprazolam, statins, cyclosporine, and tacrolimus.

TRAZODONE

Chemical Group
Triazolopyridine derivative

Trade Name
Desyrel (Apothecon)

Forms Available
Tablets of 50, 100, 150, and 300 mg

Pharmacokinetics
Half-life is 10 to 15 hours; bioavailability increased with food.

Dispensing
Once a day dosing if less than or equal to 100 mg

Range of Dosing
Adults: 150 to 400 mg per day.
Children: there is no recommended dose available. In clinical practice, starting dose is 25 mg q.h.s. It may be increased to 50 mg for sleep difficulties.
Elderly: 25 to 200 mg per day.

FDA Approval
Depression

Possible Mechanism of Action
$5HT_2$ antagonism + serotonin reuptake inhibition

Possible Advantages
Can be used in lower doses to manage sleep difficulties (it does not interfere with REM sleep pattern)

Side Effects
- Priapism
- A_1 antagonism-orthostatic hypotension
- H_1 antagonism: sedation

Drug Interactions
- May increase levels of digoxin and phenytoin.
- Amprenavir and cimetidine may increase levels of trazodone.

MIRTAZAPINE

Chemical Group
Piperazino-azepine group

Trade Name
Remeron (Organon)

Forms Available
Tablets of 15, 30, and 45 mg

Pharmacokinetics
Half-life is 20 to 40 hours; bioavailability is 80% and un-affected by food.

Dispensing
Once daily

Range of Dosing
Adults: up to 45 mg per day.
Children: optimal dose is not known.
Elderly: 7.5 to 45 mg per day.

FDA Approval
Depression

Possible Mechanism of Action
Noradrenergic and specific serotonergic antagonist (NaSSA): increases NE; increased $5HT_{1A}$ receptor stimulation; while antagonizes $5HT_2$ and $5HT_3$ receptors.

Possible Advantages
• Refractory depression/SSRI nonresponders; HIV patients, to improve appetite; anorexia nervosa; weight gain; anxious depression; no interference with sexual function; no nausea or diarrhea.
• Overall, $5HT_2$ and $5HT_3$ receptor antagonism improves tolerability of this drug.

Side Effects
H_1 antagonism causes weight gain and sedation, but also may contribute to reduction in anxiety.

Drug Interactions
Metabolized by CYP 3A4; therefore, decreased levels may occur when coprescribed with protease inhibitors, keto-conazole, erythromycin, nefazodone, and cimetidine.

BUPROPION

Chemical Group
Aminoketone group

Trade Name
Wellbutrin; Zyban (Glaxo Wellcome)

Forms Available
IR formulation available in 75- and 100-mg tablets; sustained-release (SR) formulation available in 100, 150, and 200 mg.

Pharmacokinetics
Half-life 14 hours

Dispensing
B.i.d. dosing, unless SR is used

Range of Dosing
Adults: 100 mg first day, 200 to 300 mg by fourth day, effect seen in 2 to 4 weeks.
Children: starting dose is 100 mg/day, increased up to 150 mg SR, if necessary. This dose is maintained unless the child weighs more than 150 lb.
Elderly: 75 to 225 mg per day. May be activating.

FDA Approval
Depression; smoking cessation (Zyban)

Possible Mechanism of Action
Norepinephrine reuptake inhibitor + dopamine reuptake inhibitor

Possible Advantages
- Psychomotor retardation
- Atypical depression with excess sleepiness
- Pseudodementia
- May be less likely to induce switch to mania or rapid cycling in bipolar disorder
- Less sexual dysfunction
- No orthostatic hypotension or cardiac problems
- Used for smoking cessation
- May be used for stimulant withdrawal/craving
- Used as second line drug in attention-deficit hyperactivity disorder (ADHD)

Side Effects
- Risk of seizure increases with doses over 150 mg per day or 450 mg per day IR and over 200 mg per day or 400 mg per day SR
- Contraindicated in patients with an eating disorder or seizure disorder due to increased seizure risk

Drug Interactions
- Inhibits CYP 2D6; therefore, may increase levels of pimozide, desipramine, imipramine, amitriptyline, nortriptyline, and certain antiarrhythmics.
- 14-day washout with an MAOI.

DULOXETINE
Chemical Group
Duloxetine hydrochloride

Trade Name
Cymbalta (Eli Lilly and Co.)[1]

Forms Available
Pending

Pharmacokinetics
Half-life is 10.3 hours (range, 9.2 to 19.1 hours).

Dispensing
20 mg b.i.d. with increases at intervals of no less than 1 week, 40-mg dose increments; target dose of 60 mg b.i.d.

Range of Dosing
Adults: 40 to 120 mg per day
Children: little experience with using this medication
Elderly: little experience with using this medication

Site of Action
Potent and relatively balanced inhibition of the 5HT and norepinephrine (NE) reuptake transporters; weak inhibitor of dopamine (DA) reuptake transporter

FDA Approval
Depression

Possible Mechanism of Action
Inhibition of norephedrine and serotonin (NE and 5-HT)

Possible Advantages
• Lacks significant affinity for muscarinic, histaminergic, α-adrenergic, dopaminergic, serotonergic, and opioid receptors
• May produce greater efficacy than agents acting on a single neurotransmitter system
• May benefit painful physical symptoms associated with depression
• Does not appear to cause significant elevation in blood pressure

[1] Pending; not yet available.

Side Effects
- Nausea
- Headache
- Dry mouth
- Fatigue
- Insomnia/somnolence

Pregnancy
No data available.

Drug Interactions
Duloxetine is both an inhibitor and substrate of cytochrome P450 2D6.

Mood Stabilizers

LITHIUM

Chemical Group

Monovalent cation

Trade Names and Available Forms

- Eskalith capsule—300 mg (Smith Kline, Beecham)
- Eskalith CR tablets—450 mg (Smith Kline, Beecham)
- Lithobid SR tablets—300 mg (Solvay Pharmaceuticals, Inc.)
- Lithium citrate syrup—8 mEq per mL = 300 mg (Solvay Pharmaceuticals, Inc.)
- Lithium carbonate capsules—150, 300, and 600 mg

Pharmacokinetics

Half-life is 24 hours; steady state in 5 days; reaches peak level in 2 hours with regular formulation, 4 hours with SR forms.

Dispensing

Start as t.i.d. dosing; can be given once a day after reaching a steady-state therapeutic level.

Range of Dosing

Adults: 300 mg b.i.d. or t.i.d. in adults. Start slow, raise by 300 mg every 1 to 3 days. Therapeutic level is 0.5 to 1.5 mEq per L.

Children: 10 to 30 mg per kg per day; usually begin with immediate release once a day 150 or 300 mg; gradually increase to a therapeutic level of 0.6 to 0.8 mEq per L and reassess.

Elderly: 75 to 1500 mg per day. Elderly patients often require lower lithium dosages to achieve therapeutic serum levels. They may also exhibit adverse reactions at serum levels ordinarily tolerated by younger patients. May cause cognitive side effects resembling dementia.

FDA Approval

Bipolar disorder: acute mania, maintenance

Possible Mechanism of Action

Modifying second messenger system:

- Blocks recycling of inositol phosphate from phosphoinositol phosphate (PIP_2)

- Inhibits adenylate cyclase enzyme [generates cyclic adenosine monophosphate (cAMP)], which alters G-protein interaction with neurotransmitter. This mechanism may also be responsible for side effects via pancreas, thyroid, and kidney.

Possible Advantages
- Prophylaxis to prevent recurrence (0.8 to 1.0 mEq per L).
- Moderate effect for acute treatment and prophylaxis of recurrent depressive episode
- Violence, personality disorder with mood instability: trial for 12 weeks at 0.6 to 1.2 mEq per L
- Decreases suicide risk
- May have neuroprotective effect

Side Effects
- Early, as level is rising:
  - Nausea, tremor
  - SR provides excellent bioavailability with less peak-level side effects, but has a tendency to cause diarrhea due to slower absorption in small bowel
- Common: Thirst, urination, weight gain, tremor, dermatological/acne
- GI side effects: Nausea, vomiting, anorexia, diarrhea, abdominal pain; citrate syrup may lessen these symptoms

Withdrawal Effects
Prudent to decrease by 300 mg every 2 to 4 weeks; abrupt discontinuation (less than or equal to 2 weeks) may precipitate mood episode.

RENAL
- Tuberointerstitial nephritis may occur
- Long-term effects are seen in those who take divided doses versus once a day; only slight increase in sclerotic glomeruli/atrophic tubules
- Polyuria: anti-ADH action; in long term, 50% to 70% are affected. Ten percent develop nephrogenic diabetes and produce urine more than 3 L per day. These symptoms usually improve with dosage reduction or discontinuation; rarely, may need permanent treatment with K+ sparing diuretic or amiloride
- Nephrotic syndrome: should not be given lithium again

NEUROLOGIC
- 7 to 16 Hz tremor similar to essential tremor, increased by anxiety; propranolol may help

- Benign intracranial hypertension (due to poor absorption of cerebrospinal fluid, diagnosis by fundoscopy), causing headache

COGNITIVE. Dulling effect, slowing

THYROID

- Inhibits thyroid-stimulating hormone (TSH)-responsive adenyl cyclase
- Interferes with thyroid hormones at multiple sites: iodine uptake, tyrosine iodination, release of T_3/T_4
- Timing of onset is variable

PARATHYROID. Can cause hypoparathyroidism (uncommon)

CARDIAC

- Benign: T-wave flattening
- Serious: SA block; tachycardia; clinical features include syncope and palpitation
- May require ECG monitoring

DERMATOLOGY. Acne, psoriasis, folliculitis-pruritis-hyperkeratitis

GENERAL

- Hair loss
- Weight gain: 10 kg in 20% of patients (possibly due to insulinlike effect)
- Blood: benign increase in WBC

Toxicity

The degree of toxicity can be classified as:

- Early signs—ataxia, dysarthria, lack of coordination
- Mild—occurs in the range of 1.5 to 2.0 mEq per L; most often characterized by listlessness, nausea, slurring of speech, diarrhea, and coarse tremors
- Moderate—occurs in the range of 2.0 to 2.5 mEq per L; most often characterized by coarse tremors and other CNS symptoms such as confusion or delirium, pronounced ataxia
- Severe—begins with levels at 2.5 to 3.0 mEq per L; most often characterized by significant alterations in consciousness, spontaneous attacks of hyperextension of extremities, choreoathetosis, seizures, coma, or death

With an acute overdose, treatment includes the use of various supportive measures because no antidote is available. The initial recommended steps are:

- Serum measurement of lithium, creatinine, electrolytes, and plasma osmolality

- Gastric lavage
- Monitoring of fluid intake and output
- Obtaining a history about the timing and amount of lithium taken
- A neurological exam including mental status examination and baseline EEG

Special Groups

Rapid cyclers: not as initially responsive, but may show improvement in a year

Elderly: start 300 mg b.i.d. only; glomerular filtration rate (GFR) is decreased

Pregnancy: GFR increased; may need higher levels. At parturition, there is risk of toxicity due to loss of water; Ebstein's anomaly in newborns exposed to lithium in the first trimester

Children: dysarthria, nocturnal enuresis

Metabolism and Drug Interactions

- Thiazides are absorbed at renal distal convoluted tubule. Sodium and lithium are reabsorbed at renal proximal convoluted tubule and loop only, so thiazides will increase lithium levels by 30% to 50%.
- Nonsteroidal antiinflammatory drugs (NSAIDs), angiotensin converting enzyme (ACE) inhibitors can increase lithium level.
- Coffee and theophylline can decrease lithium level.

Tests

- Serum level 12 hours after last dose: after 5 to 7 days with each dose change; when level is stable, check every 6 to 12 months
- Renal function: 24-hour pretreatment creatinine clearance; blood urea nitrogen (BUN) and serum creatinine every 6 to 12 months
- Thyroid function every 6 to 12 months
- Serum human chorionic gonadotropin (HCG) in females of child-bearing age
- Screening ECG

VALPROATE

Chemical Group
2-Propyl-pentanoic acid

Trade Name
Depacon, Depakote, Depakene (Abbott Labs)

Forms Available
- Divalproex[1] sodium delayed-release (DR) tablets—**Depakote:** 125, 250, and 500 mg
- Divalproex sodium extended-release (ER) tablets—**Depakote:** 250 and 500 mg
- Divalproex sodium-coated particles in capsules—**Depakote Sprinkles:** 125 mg
- Valproic acid—**Depakene:** 250 mg capsule and 250 mg per 5 mL syrup
- Sodium valproate—**Depacon** (injectable): 500 mg per 5 mL

Pharmacokinetics
Half-life is 8 hours for the delayed-release (DR) tablets, and 9 to 16 hours for the extended-release (ER) preparations.

Dispensing
Usually b.i.d

Range of Dosing
Adults: 250 mg t.i.d. or full-dose rapid titration with 15 to 30 mg per kg body weight and check for side effects. Adequate serum levels achieved in 2 to 3 days. Final level can be at 50 to 150 μg per mL. Depakote ER is administered as a single dose. The ER form is not bioequivalent to the DR tablets given b.i.d. because they cause 20% less fluctuation in concentration. If dosage adjustment is required in smaller doses than the ER form, then the DR forms must be used. Recommended dose for ER is 500 mg once daily for a week and then increasing to 1,000 mg once daily the next week based on tolerability and need.
Children: 15 to 20 mg per kg per day.
Elderly: 125 to 1,800 mg per day. May cause weight gain and impair concentration and recall.

FDA Approval
Bipolar disorder, acute mania; seizure disorders

[1] Divalproex = sodium valproate + valproic acid.

- Depakene—approved for monotherapy or adjunctive therapy for simple and complex absence seizures and adjunctive therapy for patients with multiple seizures, including absence seizures
- Depakote—approved for monotherapy and adjunctive therapy for complex partial seizures alone or in association with other disorders; also as monotherapy for bipolar mania
- Depacon—approved for same indications as Depakene and Depakote when injectable form is indicated

Possible Mechanism of Action
- Increases gamma-aminobutyric acid (GABA) at benzodiazepine site
- Opens chloride channel
- Synergistic action with lithium
- Inhibits protein kinase C (PKC)

Possible Advantages
- Epilepsy and mood problems
- Acute mania
- Prophylaxis for mania, depression; mixed and rapid cycling episodes may be resistant to lithium
- Cyclothymia at very low doses (125 to 500 mg per day)
- Affective disorders in developmentally disabled
- PTSD
- Migraine
- Panic disorder
- May have neuroprotective effect

Side Effects
- Hepatoxicity; thrombocytopenia; pancreatitis (idiosyncratic)
- Rash
- Weight gain, increased appetite
- Hair loss
- GI distress—nausea, vomiting, and diarrhea (less with divalproex)
- Cognitive dulling
- Pregnancy—neural tube defects ($\sim$1%)
- Possibly contributes to polycystic ovarian syndrome (PCOS)
- Most serious adverse effects: hepatic failure (primarily in the very young), pancreatitis, and teratogenicity (black box warnings)

Metabolism and Drug Interactions
- In children younger than 2 years, metabolites cause hepatic impairment

- Salicylates increase valproic acid level
- Lamotrigine level is doubled by valproic acid
- SSRIs and valproic acid mutually increase each other's levels
- Rifampin and anticonvulsants may increase valproate levels

Tests
- CBC: check for leukopenia, thromboctopenia
- Liver function test (LFT): hepatic transaminase increase
- Pancreatic enzymes

LAMOTRIGINE

Chemical Group
Phenyltriazine

Trade Name
Lamictal (Glaxo Wellcome)

Forms Available
Tablets of 25, 100, 150, and 200 mg; chewable/dispersible tablets of 2, 5, and 25 mg.

Pharmacokinetics
Half-life ~15 hours; varies depending on age and use of concomitant anticonvulsants.

Dispensing
B.i.d.; when stopping, should be withdrawn over 2 weeks

Range of Dosing
Adults: 300 to 500 mg per day; gradual dosing (25-mg increments) to prevent rash.
Children: 2 to 10 mg per kg per day. Refer to prescribing information for doses when initiating therapy; usually dosed by weekly increments of 25 to 50 mg to decrease risk of rash.
Elderly: Dose selection for the elderly should be cautious, usually starting at the low end of the dosing range.

FDA Approval
- Monotherapy for bipolar disorder, maintenance phase, depression
- Adjunctive therapy in adults with partial seizures; in pediatric and adult patients, for generalized seizures in Lennox-Gestaut syndrome
- Monotherapy in adults with partial seizures

Possible Mechanism of Action
Inhibition of voltage-sensitive sodium channels, which stabilize neuronal membranes and modulates presynaptic release of excitatory transmitters (e.g., glutamate, aspartate). Also there is possible weak inhibition of serotonin $5HT_3$ receptors.

Possible Advantages
Alternative choice for stabilizing mood
May have acute antidepressant and antimanic effects
Bipolar II, rapid cyclers

Side Effects

- Blood: WBC will usually fall if dose is increased faster than 100 mg/wk; pure red cell aplasia
- Dermatologic: in 10% of cases; rash occurs within 4 to 6 weeks, maculopapular-erythematous eruptions; serious Stevens Johnson's syndrome, toxic epidermal necrolysis, angioedema, lymphadenopathy; accumulates in melanin-containing tissues
- Hepatic failure
- GI: nausea, vomiting, and diarrhea
- Neurologic: somnolence, dizziness, ataxia, tremor, headache, diplopia, blurred vision

Metabolism and Drug Interactions

All the anticonvulsants decrease lamotrigine level except valproate, which increases levels, therefore, dose should be decreased when combined with valporate.

Other Antiepileptic Agents

CARBAMAZEPINE

Chemical Group
5H-dibenzapine-5-carboxamide

Trade Name
Tegretol (Novartis Pharmaceuticals)

Forms Available
Tablets of 200 mg; chewable tablets of 100 mg; liquid (syrup) 100 mg per 5 mL; carbatrol ER sprinkles 200 and 300-mg capsules

Pharmacokinetics
Half-life 18 to 55 hours; due to autoinduction may fall to 5 to 20 hours with repeated dosing, plateaus in 3 to 5 weeks. Peak levels in 4 to 8 hours.

Dispensing
B.i.d. or t.i.d.

Range of Dosing
Adults: 4 to 12 μg per mL, core range 6 to 10 μg per mL. Start with 200 mg b.i.d., increasing by 200-mg increments to 1,000 mg per day. Can do more rapid titration in 2 weeks. Recommended maximum dose of 1,800 mg. Check for autoinduction in 2 to 6 weeks.
Children: 10 to 30 mg per kg per day. Start at a low dose of 200 mg QHS or 200 mg b.i.d., and increase depending on the tolerability (within 1 week to 1 month) to reach therapeutic level.
Elderly: 50 to 1,200 mg per day. Can cause agranulocytosis.

FDA Approval
- Seizure disorder
  - Partial seizure with complex symptomatology
  - Generalized tonic-clonic seizures
  - Mixed seizure patterns
- Trigeminal neuralgia
- **Not approved** for bipolar disorder

Possible Mechanism of Action
Inhibits repetitive firing of action potentials by inactivating Na^+ channels. Inhibits kindling (i.e., repeated subthreshold activity that can produce epileptic activity)

Possible Advantages

Helpful in rapid cycling; takes 6 to 12 months to judge. May not decrease all affective recurrences. Helpful in acute mania, neuropathic pain, impulse control, and alcohol withdrawal

Side Effects

- Rapid dose increase: nausea, vomiting, slurred speech, dizziness, drowsiness, ataxia
- Dose related: sedation, low WBC, high LFT, ataxia, cognitive slowing (motor more than mental)
- Less dose related: tremor, cardiac conduction delay, syndrome of antidiuretic hormone (SIADH)-hyponatremia, low T_3/T_4
- Idiosyncratic: rash 10 days after (red, raised, itchy), rarely severe
- Hepatitis
- Blood dyscrasias: aplastic anemia, low WBC (less than 4,000), low platelets (less than 100,000), bone marrow toxicity

Toxicity / Overdose

(Due to rapid rise in levels) nystagmus, tremor, respiratory depression; treatment: supportive, hemodialysis not effective because highly protein bound

Pregnancy

Craniofacial defects (11%), developmental delay, neural tube defects (~1%)

Metabolism and Drug Interactions

Potent inducer of P450 system, includes autoinduction. SSRIs can inhibit carbamazepine (CBZ) metabolism.

Tests

CBC with platelets every 6 to 12 months; stop if WBC is less than 3,000, neutrophils less than 1,500 LFT, renal function testing (RFT) and thyroid function test (TFT) levels every 6 to 12 months

OXCARBAZEPINE

Chemical Name
10, 11-Dihydro-10-oxo-5-H dibenzazepine-5 carboxamide

Trade Name
Trileptal (Novartis Pharmaceuticals)

Forms Available
Tablets of 150, 300, and 600 mg; 60 mg per mL oral suspension.

Pharmacokinetics
Half-life for parent compound: 2 hours; for active metabolite: 9 hours. Reaches peak serum concentration in 2 to 3 days.

Dispensing
B.i.d. dosing

Range of Dosing
Adults: initial dose is 300 mg b.i.d.; usual daily dose is 1,200 mg per day in two divided doses. Dosage increases are made every 3 days in increments of 150 or 300 mg, depending on weight and tolerability.
Children: 8 mg per kg per day and should not exceed 600 mg per day given in two divided doses.
Elderly: start at lowest possible dose. Clinical trials have shown that oxcarbazepine in elderly patients produced maximum plasma concentrations and area under the curve (AUC) values of 10-monohydroxy metabolite (MHD) that are 30% to 60% higher than in younger patients. Age-related creatinine clearance is the cause.

FDA Approval
Adults: monotherapy or adjuvant therapy for partial seizure disorder.
Children: adjuvant therapy for partial seizure disorder, ages 4 to 16 years.

Possible Mechanism of Action
Results from parent compound, as well as MHD. MHD blocks voltage-sensitive sodium channels, stabilizing hyperexcited neuronal membranes, inhibiting repetitive firing, and decreasing the propagation of synaptic impulses. These actions are believed to prevent seizures or rage attacks and aggression.

Possible Advantages

- Rapid cycling; takes 6 to 12 months to judge
- May not decrease all affective recurrences
- May be helpful in acute mania, neuropathic pain, disorders of impulse control, alcohol withdrawal

Side Effects

- No dose adjustment is needed for hepatically impaired subjects.
- There is a linear correlation between creatinine clearance and renal clearance of MHD.
- Rapid dose increase may cause headache, nausea, vomiting, slurred speech, dizziness, drowsiness, and ataxia.
- Dose related: low sodium levels, ataxia, cognitive slowing (motor more than mental).
- Treatment of overdose: supportive; hemodialysis not helpful because 40% of MHD is protein bound.

Metabolism and Drug Interactions

Completely absorbed and extensively metabolized to MHD. It can inhibit CYP 2C19 and induce CYP 3A4/5.

Tests

CBC (leucocytopenia, thrombocytopenia); electrolytes (low potassium and sodium); serum creatinine; LFT [gamma glutamyl transferase (GGT), serum transaminases elevated].

GABAPENTIN

Chemical Group
1-(Aminomethyl) cyclohexaneacetic acid

Trade Name
Neurontin (Parke-Davis)

Forms Available
Capsules of 100, 300, and 400 mg; tablets of 600 and 800 mg; and solution 250 mg per 5 mL.

Pharmacokinetics
Half-life 5 to 9 hours, peaks in 2 to 3 hours, reaches steady state in 1 to 2 days

Dispensing
T.i.d. dosing

Range of Dosing
Adults: start as 300 mg per day, then 300 mg b.i.d. on second day, then 300 mg t.i.d. on third day. 1,800 mg per day for epilepsy and 900 to 1,500 mg per day for mood disorders in adults. Range is 200 to 3,600 mg per day.
Children: 5 to 30 mg per kg per day.
Elderly: more likely to have decreased renal function. Care should be taken in dose selection based on creatinine clearance values in these patients:
- Creatinine clearance greater than 60 mL per min = 400 mg t.i.d.
- Creatinine clearance greater than 30 to 60 mL per min = 300 mg t.i.d.
- Creatinine clearance greater than 15 to 30 mL per min = 300 mg q.i.d.

FDA Approval
Approved for adjunctive therapy of partial seizures with and without secondary generalization in adults with epilepsy and for postherpetic neuralgia.

Possible Mechanism of Action
Structurally similar to GABA, but does not act through GABA receptors. Its action is undefined and studies show that it has possible affinity for cholinergic receptors in the neurons of the brain, but not in the periphery. Possibly increases GABA in the substantia nigra as well.

Possible Advantages

- Has a lipophilic cyclohexane ring that allows it to cross blood–brain barrier. Increases GABA only in substantia nigra-increased synthesis and accumulation of GABA
- Decreased release of dopamine and adrenergic (DA), NE, 5HT
- Binding site is calcium channel subunit
- Wide therapeutic index, so blood levels are unnecessary
- Anxiolytic effect; doubtful mood stabilizing effect
- Neuropathic pain and migraine

Side Effects

- Common: somnolence, dizziness, ataxia, fatigue
- Uncommon: lowers WBC, platelets
        weight gain
        stuttering
        involuntary twitches
        hypomania
- In pregnant rats: hydronephrosis and hydroureters

Metabolism and Drug Interactions

No drug interactions; eliminated by kidneys. Cimetidine decreases renal clearance.

TIAGABINE

Chemical Group
(-)-(R)-1-[4,4-Bis(3-methyl-2-thienyl)-3- butenyl] nipecotic acid hydrochloride

Trade Name
Gabitril (Cephalon)

Forms Available
Tablets: 2, 4, 12, and 16 mg.

Pharmacokinetics
The elimination half-life is 7 to 9 hours, with peak plasma concentrations occurring at approximately 45 minutes following an oral dose, hence given with food for slower absorption. The pharmacokinetics of tiagabine are linear over the single dose range of 2 to 24 mg; after multiple dosing, steady state is achieved within 2 days.

Dispensing
B.i.d.-q.i.d. dosing

Range of Dosing
Adults: start at 4 mg per day, then increase weekly by 4 to 8 mg per day until clinical response or up to 56 mg per day dose.
Children: used only in children 12 years or older, dose range is 4 to 32 mg per day
Elderly: not known

FDA Approval
Approved for adjunctive therapy of partial seizures in adults and children 12 years and older.

Possible Mechanism of Action
Blocks sodium channels and also enhances GABA receptors.

Possible Advantages
- Potential role in treatment refractory bipolar mood disorder
- Adjunctive therapy for inadequately controlled partial epilepsy

Side Effects
- Common: dizziness, somnolence, depression, confusion, asthenia
- Uncommon: serious skin rash; EEG abonormalties and status epilepticus reported

Metabolism and Drug Interactions
Carbamazepine and phenytoin decrease levels. Tiagabine decreases valproate levels. No interaction with cimetidine.

TOPIRAMATE

Chemical Group
Sulfamate-substituted monosaccharide

Trade Name
Topamax (Ortho-McNeil Pharmaceutical)

Forms Available
Tablets of 25, 100, and 200 mg; sprinkle capsules of 15 and 25 mg.

Pharmacokinetics
Half-life less than or equal to 15 hours.

Dispensing
B.i.d. dosing

Range of Dosing
Adults: start at 50 mg per day. Increase to 400 mg per day in divided doses. Discontinue gradually.
Children: 3 to 6 mg per kg per day. For very young children, start at 25 mg per day and increase by 25 mg every other day.
Elderly: in clinical trials, no age-related difference in effectiveness or adverse reactions were seen. The possibility of age-associated renal functional abnormalities should be considered.

FDA Approval
Approved for adjunctive therapy of partial onset seizures in adults

Possible Mechanism of Action
Blocks sodium channels and also enhances GABA receptors.

Possible Advantages
Weight loss; questionable mood stabilizing and anxiolytic effects

Side Effects
- Cognitive dulling
- Confusion and memory problems
- Parathesias
- Kidney stones
- Acute myopia and secondary angle closure glaucoma
- Unknown effect in pregnancy

Metabolism and Drug Interaction

CBZ decreases topiramate levels. Oral contraceptives less effective. With valproic acid, mutual decrease in levels. Can be used in older patients. Children metabolize rapidly.

ZONISAMIDE

Chemical Group
Sulfonamide; 1–2-benzisoxazole-3-methanesulfonamide

Trade Name
Zonegran (Elan Pharmaceuticals)

Forms Available
Capsule of 100 mg.

Pharmacokinetics
Half-life of 63 hours; decreased to 24 to 63 hours with coadministration of other antiepileptics; peaks in 2 to 6 hours. Reaches steady state in 14 days.

Dispensing
Q.i.d. or b.i.d.; dose reduction or discontinuation should be done gradually

Range of Dosing
Adults: initiate therapy with 100 mg per day for 2 weeks. Increase dose by 100 mg per day every 2 weeks up to 400 mg per day. Effective range is 100 to 600 mg per day; no suggestion of increased response with doses greater than 400 mg per day.

Children: safety and efficacy younger than the age of 16 years has not been established.

Elderly: more likely to have decreased renal function and creatinine clearance; consider renal function monitoring. Increased AUC by 35% with creatinine clearance less than 20 mL per min.

FDA Approval
Adjuvant therapy in treatment of partial seizures in adults with epilepsy; **not approved** for pediatric patients younger than 16 years.

Possible Mechanism of Action
- Inhibits voltage-dependent sodium currents and T-type calcium channels to supress repetitive firing of neurons
- Blocks glutamate receptors to decrease excitation
- Enhances GABA-mediated inhibition to reduce hyperpolarization

Possible Advantages
May be neuroprotective due to decreased lipid peroxidation in cortex and decreased glutamate excitotoxicity, such

as ischemic cerebral damage. Prevents dopaminergic neurodegeneration and facilitates serotonergic neurotransmission.

Side Effects
- Allergy/hypersensitivity
- Hematological: ecchymosis, rash, pruritis, luekopenia
- Neurological: depression; psychosis; psychomotor slowing, including speech and language difficulties; confusion; fatigue; somnolence; headache; tremor; incoordination
- Kidney stones
- In pediatric patients: oligohydrosis and hyperthermia
- Teratogenic

Metabolism and Drug Interaction
Reduced to 2-sulfamoylacetyl phenol by CYP 3A4; drugs that either induce or inhibit CYP 3A4 may alter serum concentration. Excreted primarily in urine as parent compound and as the glucuronide of a metabolite.

Tests
Monitor renal function; alkaline phosphatase, BUN, and creatine clearance in renally impaired patients and elderly

Anxiolytics/Sedative-Hypnotics

BENZODIAZEPINES

Chemical Group

Benzodiazepines, example: 8-chloro-1-methyl-6-phenyl-4H—s-triazolo[4,3-a][1,4]benzodiazepine(alprazolam)

Trade Names

Refer to Table 7-1 for trade names.

Pharmacokinetics

Due to different chemical structures, benzodiazepines (BZDs) vary in their pharmacokinetic properties (Table 7-2).

Dispensing

Refer to Table 7-1 for dispensing information.

Range of Dosing

Refer to Table 7-1 for dose ranges.

Possible Mechanism of Action

- Bind to a specific site on $GABA_A$ receptors
- Linked to, but distinct from, the GABA receptor recognition site
- Enhances GABA recognition potentiating inhibitory action

Possible Advantages

- Wide range of selection (Table 7-1) to benefit individual patient, minimizing adverse effects due to different pharmacokinetic properties
- Effective in several anxiety and sleep disorders, as well as anxiety and agitation associated with other disorders
- Safe in overdose if used alone

Side Effects

- Sedation—initially, but often subsides as anxiolytic action sets in
- Behavioral disinhibition
- Psychomotor impairment—coordination and sustained attention

Table 7-1.   Commonly used benzodiazepines

	Generic Name	Trade Name	Half-life, Including Metabolite (hr)	Lipid Solubility	Active Metabolite	Dose Range
Intermediate to long acting	Diazepam[a]	Valium	20–70	High	Yes	5–100 mg/d
	Lorazepam[a]	Ativan	10–70	Moderate	No	1–6 mg/d
	Clonazepam[a]	Klonopin	19–50	Moderate	No	1–6 mg/d
Short to intermediate acting	Alprazolam[a]	Xanax	8–15	Moderate	No	0.5–6 mg/d
	Oxazepam[a]	Serax	5–15	Moderate	No	5–60 mg/d
	Temazepam[b]	Restoril	8–12	High	No	15–45 mg/d
	Midazolam[a]	Versed	1.5–3.5	High	No	5–15 mg/ivdose

[a]Most frequently used as anxiolytic.
[b]Most frequently used as hypnotic.

**Table 7-2. Pharmacokinetic properties
of benzodiazepines**

Properties	Short Acting	Long Acting
Potency	High	Low
Daily dosage frequency	Q4–6 hr	b.i.d. or once daily
Interdose anxiety	Frequent	Rare
Accumulation	Little or none	Common
Hypnotic hangover effects	None or mild	Mild to moderate
Rebound anxiety	Frequent	Infrequent
Dependency risk	High	Low
Onset withdrawal symptoms	1–3 d	4–7 d
Duration withdrawal symptoms	2–5 d	8–15 d
Paradoxical effects	Frequent	Infrequent
Anterograde amnesia	Frequent	Infrequent
Intramuscular administration	Rapid absorption	Slow absorption
IV risk	Low	High with rapid injection
Active metabolites	None or few	Many

Source: Adapted from Janicak PG, Davis JM, Perskorn SH, et al.
Principles and practice of psychopharmacotherapy, 3rd ed. Philadelphia: Lippincott Williams & Wilkins, 2001.

- Cognitive impairment—even with a single dose
- Confusion, ataxia, excitement, agitation, transient hy-
potension, vertigo, and GI distress in some patients
- Psychological dependence

Withdrawal Symptoms
Although BZDs can produce dependence, hence withdrawal symptoms, this is unlikely with short-term use.
Withdrawal is more likely when higher potency BZDs are
taken for a longer duration and discontinued abruptly.

Symptoms
- Various GI symptoms
- Diaphoresis
- Tremor, lethargy, dizziness, headaches
- Increased acuity for smell and sound
- Restlessness, insomnia, irritability, anxiety
- Tinnitus

- Feelings of depersonalization
- Seizures, especially with abrupt withdrawal of high potency BZD (e.g., alprazolam)

Tapering

It is important to taper the BZD dose to avoid withdrawal symptoms. Necessary in patients who have taken a BZD for more than 4 months, especially with potent, short-acting BZD. History of seizures is another important reason to slowly taper BZD.

BUSPIRONE

Chemical Group
Azospirocanedione

Trade Name
Buspar (Bristol Myers-Squibb)

Forms Available
Tablets of 5, 10, and 15 mg, 30 mg (scored)

Pharmacokinetics
Half-life 5 to 11 hours; bioavailability increased with food

Dispensing
T.i.d. dosing

Range of Dosing
Adults: start with 5 mg t.i.d.; maximum effect in 4 to 6 weeks; can be discontinued abruptly.
Children: the very young can begin at 2.5 mg t.i.d. and increase to 5 mg t.i.d. Given at 0.2 to 1 mg per kg per day.
Elderly: start at 5 mg b.i.d., may increase to maximum of 60 mg per day. Anxiolytic effect at low dose unpredictable; modest agitation effects at higher doses.

FDA Approval
Generalized anxiety disorder (GAD)

Possible Mechanism of Action:
- $5HT_{1a}$ receptor partial agonist: decreases 5HT turnover
- 1-Phenyl-piperazine metabolite—acts via α_2 adrenergic receptors, increase firing rate in locus caeruleus.

Possible Advantages
No dependency problems, sedation, or psychomotor retardation; safe in overdose.

Side Effects
- Headache, GI distress, dizziness
- Less useful in those who have been on BZDs

Drug Interactions
- Avoid use with MAOIs
- Inhibitors of CYP 3A4, such as grapefruit juice, diltiazem, erythromycin, and itraconazole, may elevate levels of buspirone

ZOLPIDEM

Chemical Group
Imidazopyridine

Trade Name
Ambien (Searle)

Forms Available
Tablets: 5 and 10 mg

Pharmacokinetics
Half-life 2.4 hours in adults; rapidly absorbed after oral administration, high plasma protein binding capacity; peak blood levels reached in 2.2 hours; 6 to 8 hours of duration of action.

Dispensing
Once daily QHS.

Range of Dosing
Adults: 2.5 to 10 mg immediately before bedtime. Maximum dose recommended is 20 mg.
Children: no information available.
Elderly: 2.5 to 5 mg immediately before bedtime, maximum dose should not exceed 10 mg. Insufficient data to conclude that cognitive function is not impaired in the elderly.

FDA Approval
Short-term treatment of insomnia

Possible Mechanism of Action
Nonbenzodiazepine hypnotic, which acts selectively on the alpha-subunit of the GABA-BZ receptor complex. Modulation of these chloride receptor channels potentiates the inhibitory effect of GABA.

Possible Advantages
- No muscle relaxant, anxiolytic, or anticonvulsant effects with sedative dose
- Less likely to affect sleep architecture
- No or minimal rebound withdrawal effects
- Less abuse potential than with BZDs

Side Effects

1% to 10%

- CNS: headache, drowsiness, dizziness
- Gastrointestinal: nausea, diarrhea, and vomiting
- Neuromuscular and skeletal: myalgia; less than 1%— amnesia, confusion, falls, tremor
- Appears to cause memory impairment

Metabolism and Drug Interactions

- Metabolized in liver; therefore, dose adjustment required in hepatic impairment and elderly.
- Increased effect or toxicity with alcohol, CNS depressants, and SSRIs.
- Contraindicated during lactation

ZALEPLON

Chemical Group
Pyrazolopyrimidine derivative

Trade Name
Sonata (Wyeth-Ayerst)

Form Available
Capsules: 5 and 10 mg

Pharmacokinetics
Half-life is 1 hour; rapid onset with peak effect and peak serum concentration reached within 1 hour. Duration of action 6 to 8 hours. Absorption is rapid and almost complete with 30% bioavailability. High-fat meal can prolong absorption.

Dispensing
Once daily, immediately before bedtime or when patient cannot fall asleep.

Range of Dosing
Adults: 10 mg QHS; usual dose range is 5 to 20 mg.
Children: no information available.
Elderly: 5 mg QHS.

FDA Approval
Short-term treatment of insomnia

Possible Mechanism of Action
Nonbenzodiazepine hypnotic, which acts selectively at omega-1 receptors on the alpha-subunit of the GABA-BZ receptor complex. Modulation of these chloride receptor channels potentiates the inhibitory effect of GABA.

Possible Advantages
- Decreases sleep latency with minimal effect on sleep stages.
- Due to its very short half-life, it is useful in patients with difficulty falling asleep, staying asleep, and going back to sleep after waking up at night.
- At recommended dosage, cognitive and psychomotor skills are apparantly not significantly impaired.
- Possible absence of rebound insomnia and withdrawal symptoms on discontinuation.

Side Effects

More than 10%:

- CNS: headache

1% to 10%:

- Cardiovascular system (CVS): peripheral edema
- CNS: amnesia, anxiety, depersonalization, hallucinations, somnolence, vertigo, depression, impaired coordination, dizziness, tremor
- Skin: rash, photosensitivity
- Gastrointestinal tract (GIT): abdominal pain, anorexia, colitis, dyspepsia, nausea, constipation
- Neuromuscular: myalgia, weakness

Caution: When used in patients:

- With depression, particularly with suicidal risk
- With history of drug dependence
- Performing tasks requiring mental alertness, such as operating heavy machinery or driving

Metabolism and Drug Interaction

- Zaleplon is primarily metabolized by aldehyde/oxidase and to a lesser extent by CYP 3A4. All metabolites are pharmacologically inactive.
- Zaleplon potentiates CNS effects of alcohol, imipramine, and thioridazine. Alternative drug is chosen if patient is taking CYP 3A4 inducers, such as phenytoin, carbamazepine, and phenobarbital. Lower doses of zaleplon are used when coprescribed with cimetidine (because cimetidine inhibits both aldehyde oxidase and CYP 3A4).

Adjuvant Medications

CLONIDINE

Chemical Group
Imidazoline

Trade Name
Catapres (Boehringer-Ingelheim)

Forms Available
Patches: 0.1 mg per day per week
0.2 mg per day per week
0.3 mg per day per week
Tablets: 0.1, 0.2, and 0.3 mg

Pharmacokinetics
Half-life 9 hours; peaks in 1 to 3 hours.

Dispensing
B.i.d. dosing. Tablet must be split first and must be used
0.05 mg b.i.d.

Range of Dosing
Adults: 0.1 mg b.i.d. to t.i.d. is safe. Always consider tapering the dose.
Children: start at 0.05 mg per day or b.i.d., depending on
weight and severity of problem. Titrate during week one
to a maximum of 0.1 mg t.i.d.
Elderly: start at low end of dose range, can be increased
to adult levels. Clonidine has few metabolic and serious
side effects. Has a relatively low cost, which may make
it a useful choice for the elderly. Hypotension is a possibility.

FDA Approval
Hypertension

Possible Mechanism of Action
Centrally acting, alpha-agonist

Possible Advantages
• Opioid withdrawal: decreases autonomic hyperarousal
• Gilles de la Tourette's syndrome: 2 to 3 months to assess
  benefit; 0.1 to 0.3 mg per day
• Akathisia: 0.1 to 0.2 mg per day

- First used for tics, then for ADHD, PTSD, to induce sleep, autonomic nervous system (ANS) hyperarousal
- Safe up to 0.1 mg t.i.d.

Side Effects
- Sedation
- Hypotension
- Rebound hypertension (tolerance may develop in 2 weeks)
- Dry mouth, eyes
- Nausea
- Impotence
- Postural dizziness
- Vivid dreams
- Insomnia
- Anxiety/depression
- Idiosyncratic side effects: rash, pruritus, gynecomastia
- Children develop allergy to patches; cream can help

Metabolism and Drug Interactions
- Lipophilic, penetrates blood–brain barrier
- 50% excreted by kidneys, 50% by liver
- Tricyclics can decrease the effect of clonidine

GUANFACINE

Chemical Group
Acetamide hydrochloride

Trade Name
Tenex (Robins)

Forms Available
Tablets: 1 and 2 mg

Pharmacokinetics
Half-life is 10 to 30 hours; younger patients have shorter half-life (13 to 14 hours); older patients have half-life at upper end of range.

Dispensing
Q.i.d.

Range of Dosing
Adults: recommended initial dose of 1 mg per day; maximum dose of 4 mg per day
Children: recommended maximum dose is 3 mg per day
Elderly: dose adjustment is not required. Age reduction in urinary excretion and renal clearance were observed in the elderly and accompanied by an increase in proportion of metabolites. Based on these studies and dual renal and nonrenal clearance, the dose usually does not need to be adjusted.

FDA Approval
Hypertension

Possible Mechanism of Action
Centrally acting antihypertensive with α_2 adrenoreceptor agonist action

Possible Advantages
- Opioid withdrawal: decreases autonomic hyperarousal
- Gilles de la Tourette's syndrome: 2 to 3 months to assess benefit; 0.1 to 0.3 mg per day
- Akathisia: 0.1 to 0.2 mg per day
- Given the longer half-life, midday dose can be avoided (unlike clonidine)

Side Effects
- Sedation
- Hypotension
- Dry mouth, eyes

- Nausea
- Impotence
- Postural dizziness
- Vivid dreams
- Insomnia
- Anxiety/depression
- Rebound hypertension (delayed compared with clonidine, consistent with its longer half-life)

Metabolism and Drug Interactions
- Guanfacine and its metabolites are excreted primarily in urine
- ~50% of dose eliminated in urine unchanged
- Increased sedation when given with other CNS depressant drugs

Psychostimulants

METHYLPHENIDATE

Chemical Group
Piperidine derivative

Trade Name
Ritalin (Novartis)

Forms Available
Tablets: 5, 10, and 20 mg, 20 mg SR (SR only as Ritalin, not generic).

Pharmacokinetics
Half-life is 2 to 3 hours; peaks in 1.5 to 2.5 hours. Entirely excreted in urine in 12 to 24 hours. Behavioral effects occur within 30 to 60 minutes; peak in 1 to 3 hours; dissipates in 3 to 5 hours. SR effects are seen in 1 to 2 hours; peak in 3 to 5 hours; lasts for 8 hours.

Dispensing
Usually 8 a.m., noon, and 4 p.m., if required.

Range of Dosing
Children: lower doses (0.3 mg per kg) were believed to be most helpful for learning, whereas higher doses were found to be better for social behavior. Maximum dosing is 1 mg per kg. There are significant differences in response across individuals. A safe maximum dose is 40 to 60 mg per day.
Adults: 0.5 mg per kg body weight.
Elderly: no information available.

FDA Approval
ADHD, narcolepsy

Possible Mechanism of Action
Enhances release of dopamine and to a lesser extent norepinephrine

Possible Advantages
- Improves vigilance, impulse control, fine motor coordination, and reaction time
- Reduces task irrelevant responses and improves persistence

- Reduces aggression, impulsive behavior, noisiness, non-compliance, and disruptiveness
- Improves quality of social interactions with peers, parents, and teachers

Side Effects
- Decreased appetite, sleeplessness, anxiety/irritability/crying (mood symptoms may be associated with the disorder). May be more evident in the washout time rather than in the peak plasma level period
- Stomachaches/headaches may be reported, but tend to be mild
- Tics in 1%, exacerbated in 13%
- Behavioral rebound
- Concerns about drug dependence, height and weight suppression, and heart problems are not supported by existing data

Metabolism and Drug Interactions
- Mainly metabolized to ritalanic acid and is pharmacologically inactive
- Cumulative effect with other stimulant medications and MAOIs

Tests
Baseline ECG

CONCERTA EXTENDED RELEASE

Chemical Group
Methylphenidate hydrochloride, piperadine derivative

Trade Name
Concerta (Alza Pharmaceuticals)

Forms Available
Tablets: 18, 26, 36, and 54 mg

Pharmacokinetics
Half-life is 12 hours. Initial peak level is reached in 1 to 2 hours and gradually increases over the next few hours. Peak plasma level is reached in 6 to 8 hours. Concerta uses osmotic pressure to deliver methylphenidate at a controlled rate. The tablet has an osmotically active trilayer core surrounded by a semipermeable membrane with an immediate release drug overcoat. There is a laser-drilled orifice on the push layer (outer layer of the trilayer core) at the drug layer end of the tablet. As water enters the tablet in the stomach, methylphenidate is released from the tablet through the orifice. The membrane controls the osmotic rate and drug delivery.

Dispensing
Single a.m. dosing. No evidence of dose dumping with food.

- 15 mg per day of regular tablets of methylphenidate, or 20 mg SR
- 30 mg per day of regular tablets of methylphenidate, or 40 mg SR
- 45 mg per day of regular tablets of methylphenidate, or 60 mg SR

Range of Dosing
Children: lower doses (0.3 mg per kg) were believed to help the most for learning, whereas higher doses were found to be better for social behavior. Maximum dosing is 1 mg per kg per day. There are significant differences in response across individuals. It has not been studied for children younger than 6 years of age.
Adults: 0.5 mg per kg body weight
Elderly: no information available.

FDA Approval
ADHD

Possible Mechanism of Action

Enhances norepinephrine and dopamine release; more effect on dopamine than d-amphetamine

Possible Advantages

Single dose resulting in smooth effect throughout the day; there is no need to take it at school or work

Side Effects

Headache, abdominal pain, nausea, loss of appetite, tremors, tics, high blood pressure, insomnia

Contraindications

Tics, anxiety/agitation, glaucoma

Metabolism and Drug Interactions

- Mainly metabolized to ritalanic acid, which is pharmacologically inactive
- Additive effects with other stimulant medications and MAOIs

Tests

Baseline ECG, CBC, complete metabolic profile (CMP)

METADATE CONTROLLED DELIVERY

Chemical Group
Methylphenidate HCL, piperidine derivative

Trade Name
Metadate CD (Celltech Pharmaceuticals, Inc.)

Form Available
Capsules of 20 mg

Pharmacokinetics
Methylphenidate HCL, ER capsules. The Diffucaps technology was used. The capsules contain two kinds of beads: the IR and ER beads. Thirty percent of the dose (6 mg) is provided by the IR beads and 70% of the dose (14 mg) by the ER beads. The continued release beads each have an additional ethyl cellulose coating that provides ER characteristics. The first peak plasma level is reached in 1.5 hours. Second peak is reached in 4.5 hours. The beads contain an aqueous outer protective membrane in addition to the release control membrane in ER beads. Half-life is 6.8 hours.

Dispensing
Single a.m. dosing before breakfast.

Range of Dosing
Children: start at 20 mg. Raise dose only in 20-mg increments; never more than 60 mg q.a.m. Conversion is equivalent to standard form of methylphenidate
Adults: 0.5 to 1 mg per kg body weight.
Elderly: no information available.

FDA Approval
ADHD

Possible Mechanism of Action
Enhances release of dopamine and to a lesser extent norepinephrine

Possible Advantages
- Single extended release dosing
- Long-term effects and efficacy not yet tested

Side Effects
- Decreased appetite, sleeplessness, anxiety/irritability/crying (mood symptoms may be associated with the disorder)

- Stomach aches/headaches may be reported, but tend to be mild
- Elevated blood pressure
- Behavioral rebound
- Concerns about drug dependence, height and weight suppression, and heart problems are not supported by existing data

Contraindications

Tics, anxiety/agitation, glaucoma

Metabolism and Drug Interactions

- Mainly metabolized to ritalanic acid, which is pharmacologically inactive
- Additive effects with other stimulant medications and MAOIs
- Fruit juices and ascorbic acid decrease absorption

Tests

Baseline ECG, CBC, CMP

DEXMETHYLPHENIDATE

Chemical Group
This is the d- or "right-handed" isomer of the racemic mixture found in d,1-methylphenidate. The active isomer is isolated as dexmethylphenidate.

Trade Name
Focalin (Novartis)

Forms Available
Tablets: 2.5, 5, and 10 mg

Pharmacokinetics
Half-life is 2–5 hours. Reaches peak in 1 to 4 hours. Entirely excreted in urine within 12 to 24 hours. Behavioral effects occur within 30 to 60 minutes; peak in 1 to 4 hours; dissipate in 3 to 5 hours.

Dispensing
Usually b.i.d. dosing, at least 4 hours apart

Range of Dosing
Children: starting dose is 2.5 mg. Maximum recommended dose is 20 mg per day. Patients being switched from methylphenidate should be started at half their final methylphenidate dose because it is more active.
Adults: 0.5 mg per kg per day.
Elderly: no information available.

FDA Approval
ADHD

Possible Mechanism of Action
Enhances dopamine and to a lesser extent norepinephrine release

Possible Advantages
- Improves vigilance, impulse control, fine motor coordination, and reaction time
- Reduces task-irrelevant responses and improves persistence
- Reduces aggression, impulsive behavior, noisiness, noncompliance, and disruptiveness
- Improves quality of social interactions with peers, parents, and teachers
- Efficacy is considered superior to methylphenidate because it is the active isomer

Side Effects

- Decreased appetite, sleeplessness, anxiety/irritability/crying (mood symptoms may be associated with the disorder). May be more problematic in the washout than in the peak period
- Stomach aches/headaches may be reported, but tend to be mild
- Tics in 1%, exacerbated in 13%
- Behavioral withdrawal rebound
- Concerns about drug dependence, height and weight suppression, and heart problems are not supported by existing data

Metabolism and Drug Interactions

- Mainly metabolized to ritalanic acid, which is pharmacologically inactive
- Additive effect with other stimulant medications and MAOIs

Tests

Baseline ECG

DEXTROAMPHETAMINE

Chemical Group
dextroamphetamine sulfate

Trade Name
Dexedrine (tablets and spansules) (Smith-Kline-Beecham)
DextroStat (tablets) (Shire Richwood, Inc.)

Forms Available
Dexedrine—tablets 5, 10, and 15 mg; Dexedrine spansule—capsules of 5, 10, and 15 mg; elixir 5 mg per 5 mL; DextroStat—tablets of 5 and 10 mg.

Pharmacokinetics
Half-life is 4 to 6 hours. Reaches peak in 1.5 to 2.5 hours. Behavioral effects occur within 30 to 60 minutes; peak in 1 to 3 hours; dissipated in 4 to 6 hours. Dexedrine spansule peaks in 8 to 10 hours.

Dispensing
Usually 8 a.m., noon, and 4 p.m., if required

Range of Dosing
Children: lower doses (0.15 mg per kg) were believed to be better for learning, whereas higher doses were found to be better for social behavior. Maximum dosing is 1.5 mg per kg per day. Safe maximum dose is 30 mg per day. There are significant differences in response across individuals.
Adults: 0.25 to 0.5 mg per kg body weight.
Elderly: no dose recommendations available. Some physicians see benefits as an antidepressant for elderly patients who cannot tolerate the side effects of traditional therapy. Benefits are usually noted within 36 hours and habituation is generally not a problem.

FDA Approval
ADHD, narcolepsy

Possible Mechanism of Action
Sympathomimetic that enhances norepinephrine and dopamine release.

Possible Advantages
- Improves vigilance, impulse control, fine motor coordination, and reaction time
- Reduces task irrelevant responses and improves persistence

- Reduces aggression, impulsive behavior, noisiness, non-compliance, and disruptiveness
- Improves quality of social interactions with peers, parents, and teachers

Side Effects

- Decreased appetite, sleeplessness, anxiety/irritability/crying (mood symptoms may be associated with the disorder). May be more problematic in the washout than in the peak period
- Stomach aches/headaches may be reported, but tend to be mild
- Tics in 1%, exacerbated in 13%
- Behavioral rebound
- Concerns about drug dependence, height and weight suppression, and heart problems are not supported by existing data

Metabolism and Drug Interactions

- Mainly metabolized to benzoic acid in liver; excreted in urine within 24 hours.
- Additive effect with other stimulant medications and MAOIs

Tests

Baseline ECG

PEMOLINE
Chemical Group
Oxazolidine

Trade Name
Cylert (Abbott Labs)

Forms Available
Tablets: 18.75, 37.5, and 75 mg; chewable tablets: 37.5 mg.

Pharmacokinetics
Half-life is 7 to 8 hours in children compared with 11 to 13 hours in adults. Reaches peak plasma levels in 2 to 4 hours post ingestion. Half-life increases with chronic use, which explains the delay in behavioral effects for up to 3 to 4 weeks after starting.

Dispensing
Once per day in the a.m.

Range of Dosing
Children: between 0.5 and 2 mg per kg per day or a total dose range of 18.75 to 112.5 mg per day.
Adults: no information available.
Elderly: no information available.

FDA Approval
ADHD

Possible Mechanism of Action
A sympathomimetic

Possible Advantages
No addictive potential

Side Effects
Pemoline has been associated with chemical hepatitis, which may not be irreversible in up to 3% of children taking this drug. (Refer to "Test" section below.)

Metabolism and Drug Interactions
• Within 24 hours, 50% to 70% is excreted in urine. May develop resistance to this drug; could be due to

autoinduction, other stresses, or alteration in the
dopamine receptors
- Less effect on blood pressure and heart rate

Tests

Liver function tests every 2 weeks

ADDERALL

Chemical Group
Stimulant: dextroamphetamine sulfate and amphetamine sulfate with the dextroisomer of amphetamine saccharate and d,1-amphetamine aspartate.

Trade Name
Adderall, Adderall XR (Shire Richwood, Inc.)

Forms Available
Tablets: 5, 10, 20, and 30 mg; XR in capsules: 5, 10, 15, 20, 25, and 30 mg.

Pharmacokinetics
Half-life is 2 to 3 hours; peaks in 1.5 to 2.5 hours. Entirely excreted in urine by 12 to 24 hours. Behavioral effects occur within 30 to 60 minutes; peak in 1 to 3 hours; dissipate in 3 to 5 hours. Peaks in 3 to 5 hours and lasts for 8 hours. Adderall XR peaks in 3 hours and takes 7 hours to reach maximum plasma concentration. Adderall XR contains two kinds of beads designed to give a double-pulsed delivery of amphetamine. Opening the capsule and sprinkling the contents on apple sauce results in comparable absorption to the intact capsule taken in the fasted state. Sprinkle form must be consumed immediately and must not be chewed. Food prolongs the T_{max} by 2.5 hours.

Dispensing
Usually 8 a.m. and 3 p.m., if required

Range of Dosing
Children: older than 3 years, range is between 2.5 and 30 mg per day, depending on age, weight, and response. Weight calculated dose is 0.15 to 0.2 mg per kg, or a maximum of 40 mg per day. Adderall XR recommended maximum dose is 30 mg per day.
Adults: 0.25 to 0.5 mg per kg per day
Elderly: no information available.

FDA Approval
ADHD, narcolepsy

Possible Mechanism of Action
Enhances norepinephrine and dopamine release

Possible Advantages
• Improves vigilance, impulse control, fine motor coordination, and reaction time

- Reduces task-irrelevant responses and improves persistence
- Reduces aggression, impulsive behavior, noisiness, noncompliance, and disruptiveness
- Improves quality of social interactions with peers, parents, and teachers
- May be superior in efficacy to other amphetamines

Side Effects
- Tachycardia and elevation of blood pressure
- Decreased appetite, sleeplessness, anxiety/irritability/crying (mood symptoms may be associated with the disorder)
- Stomachaches/headaches are reported, but tend to be mild
- Tics in 1%, exacerbated in 13%
- Behavioral rebound
- Concerns about drug dependence, height and weight suppression, and heart problems are not supported by existing data

Metabolism and Drug Interactions
- Mainly metabolized to ritalanic acid, which is pharmacologically inactive
- Additive effect with other stimulant medications and MAOIs
- Fruit juices and ascorbic acid decrease absorption

Tests
Baseline ECG

ATOMOXETINE

Chemical Group
Benzenepropanamine, N-methyl-gamma-(2-methylphenoxy)-, hydrochloride

Trade Name
Strattera (Eli Lilly)

Forms Available
Capsule: 10, 18, 25, 40, and 60 mg

Pharmacokinetics
Half-life is 5 hours. Peak level is reached in 1 to 2 hours after dosing. Well absorbed after oral administration. Ninety-eight percent is primarily bound to albumin in plasma. Pharmacokinetic values were similar in adults and children older than 6 years when doses were normalized to a mg per kg basis.

Dispensing
Once daily or divided dose in morning and late afternoon or early evening with food or without food. Nausea/GI complaints may be reduced when given with food.

Range of Dosing
Adults: start at 40 mg per day. Dose can be increased after minimum of 3 days and after 2 to 4 weeks if no optimal response is seen. Usual range is 60 to 120 mg per day with a mean dose of 95 mg per day, given in divided doses.

Children and adolescents (up to 70 kg body weight): start with 0.5 mg per kg per day. Dose can be increased after minimum of 3 days 1.2 to 1.4 mg per kg per day or 100 mg, whichever is less.

Children and adolescents (more than 70 kg body weight): same as adults.

Elderly: no information available.

FDA Approval
For ADHD in adults and children older than 6 years

Possible Mechanism of Action
Selective inhibition of presynaptic norepinephrine transporter

Possible Advantages
It is equipotent to methylphenidate. Further advantages need to be established.

Table 9-1. Most commonly used psychostimulants

Brand Name	Generic	Form	Dosage (mg)	Delivery System
Adderall XR	Mixed salts—dextroamphetamine and amphetamine	Capsule	5, 15, 10, 20, 25, 30	Once daily or b.i.d. dosing. Bead delivery system with double-pulsed delivery. Peak is 3 hr, but maximum plasma concentration is 7 hr.
Ritalin[a]	Methylphenidate HCL	Tablet	5, 10, 20	Immediate release b.i.d. or t.i.d. dosing Peaks in 1.9 hr
Ritalin SR[b]	Methylphenidate HCL	Tablet (sustained release)	20	Once per day or b.i.d. Effect lasts 8–12 hr Peaks in 4.7 hr
Ritalin LA	Methylphenidate HCL	Capsule (extended release)	20, 30, 40	Bimodal release profile, once per day dosing.
Dexedrine	Dextroamphetamine	Tablet, Spanule, and elixir	5, 10, 15 mg; 5 mg per mL	b.i.d. or t.i.d. dosing Effect seen with in 30 to 60 min. Peak 1–3 hr with tablets. Peak 8 to 10 hr for spanules
Methylin	Methylphenidate HCL	Tablet	5, 10, 20	Immediate release b.i.d. or t.i.d. dosing Peaks in 1.9 hr

Methylin ER	Methylphenidate HCL	Tablet (extended release)	10, 20	b.i.d. or t.i.d. dosing Effect lasts 8 hr Peaks in 4.7 hr
Metadate ER	Methylphenidate HCL	Tablet (extended release)	10, 20	b.i.d. or t.i.d. dosing Effect lasts 8 hr
Metadate CD	Methylphenidate HCL	Diffucaps—bead delivery system	20	Bead delivery system Once per day or b.i.d. Effect lasts 8–12 hr Peaks in 2–4 hr
Concerta	Methylphenidate HCL	Tablet (extended release)	18, 36, 54	Osmotic pressure Once per day or b.i.d. Effect lasts 12 hr. Peaks in 6 hr.
Cylert	Methylphenidate HCL	Tablet	18.75, 37.5, 75	Once per day a.m. dose Peaks in 2–4 hr
Provigil	Modafinil	Tablet	100, 200	
Focalin	D-isomer of methyl-phenidate	Tablet	2.5, 5, 10	b.i.d. dosing Peaks in 1–4 hr

[a]Ritalin 5 mg ~ Concerta 18 mg.
[b]Ritalin SR 20 mg ~ Concerta 18 mg; Ritalin SR, Metadate ER (bioequivalent).
Source: Adapted from a version of the table developed by Esparanza Salinas, MD.

Side Effects

Most common side effects include dyspepsia, headache, nausea, fatigue, decreased appetite, dizziness, insomnia, and mood swings. It may impair sexual function in adults with erectile disturbance and impotence.

Metabolism and Drug Interactions

Metabolized by CYP 2D6; drugs that inhibit CYP 2D6 such as fluoxetine, paroxetine, and quinidine can increase atomoxetine level.

Caution

Must be used cautiously with pressor agents, given the possibility of increased blood pressure. The capsule should not be broken and sprinkled on food (may cause irritation of mucosa and skin).

Contraindications

Atomoxetine should not be administered with or within 2 weeks of MAOI administration. Atomoxetine use with IV albuterol is contraindicated.

See Table 9-1 for most commonly used psychostimulants.

Drug Therapy for Substance Use Disorders

NALTREXONE

Chemical Group
Synthetic congener of oxymorphone (phenanthrene-containing opioid)

Trade Name
Nalorex, Revia (Dupont)

Forms Available
Tablets: 50 mg

Pharmacokinetics
Half-life of 4 hours; peak plasma level in 1 hour. Fifty mg of naltrexone can block the pharmacological effects of 25 mg of IV heroin for 24 hours. One hundred mg and 150 mg of naltrexone are effective for 48 and 72 hours, respectively.

Dispensing
QD dosing

Range of Dosing
Alcoholism: 50 mg daily
Opioid dependence: Verify that patient has not used opioids in the last 7 to 10 days prior to initiating therapy. Confirmation is through urine analysis for opioids and/or a naloxone challenge test. Start therapy with an initial dose of 25 mg. If no signs of opiate withdrawal, then 50 mg per day thereafter. Alternative dosing schedules:

- 50 mg every weekday with 100 mg every Saturday
- 100 mg every other day
- 150 mg every third day

FDA Approval
Alcoholism (suppress cravings); opioid addiction (blocks effects of exogenously administered opioids)

Possible Mechanism of Action
Competitive blockade at CNS opiate receptors

Possible Advantages
- No development of tolerance or dependence
- Blocks physical dependence to heroin or morphine when coadministered with these agents

Side Effects
- Dose-related hepatotoxicity
- In alcoholism: nausea, headache, dizziness, anxiety, fatigue, insomnia, vomiting
- In opioid addiction: joint pain, muscle pain, abdominal pain/cramps, nausea, anxiety, vomiting, fatigue, rash, sexual dysfunction
- Opioid withdrawal symptoms may occur

Metabolism and Drug Interactions
Extensive hepatic first-pass metabolism (bioavailability ranging from 5% to 40%) to form 6-beta-naltrexol. Primarily excreted in urine.

- More severe liver damage when used with other hepatotoxic agents, such as disulfiram
- Interaction with thioridazine causes increased somnolence and fatigue
- Decreased effectiveness of opioid-containing medications (e.g., cough syrups, antidiarrheals, opioid analgesics)

Contraindications/Cautions
- Patients receiving opioid analgesics or currently taking opioids
- Patients in acute opioid withdrawal
- Acute hepatitis or liver failure
- Nursing mothers
- Safety and efficacy are yet to be established in patients younger than 18 years of age

Tests
Liver function tests

METHADONE

Chemical Group
3-Heptan-1, 6-dimethylamino-4,4-diphenyl hydrochloride

Trade Name
Dolophine (Abbott)

Forms Available
Tablets: 5 and 10 mg; diskets: 40 mg; injections: 10 mg per mL.

Pharmacokinetics
Plasma half-life is 15 hours; peak plasma level in 4 hours

Dispensing
Q.i.d. or divided daily doses as needed

Range of Dosing
Adults: For severe pain: 2.5 to 10 mg every 3 to 4 hours as needed
For detoxification treatment: Initially, 15 to 40 mg once daily for 3 days; then decrease to q.i.d. or QOD. Higher doses may be needed for more severe physical dependency. Amount should always be enough to control withdrawal symptoms. Treatment duration longer than 21 days indicates progression from detoxification to maintenance treatment. Maintenance amount varies; maximum is 120 mg per day.
Children: not advised for patients younger than 18 years of age
Elderly: should be started on lower doses.

FDA Approval
Detoxification (treatment of withdrawal syndrome) from opiate addiction, severe pain

Possible Mechanism of Action
Acts at CNS mu opiate receptor agonist, mimicking the action of morphine, suppressing the opiate withdrawal symptoms, and responsible for analgesic effect.

Possible Advantages
• Less addiction potential
• Long-acting agent
• Does not cause euphoria

Side Effects
• Respiratory depression
• Hypotension

- Dizziness and light-headedness
- Nausea and vomiting
- Sweating
- Sedation, dysphoria, and euphoria
- Constipation and urinary retention
- Decreased libido

Metabolism and Drug Interactions

Metabolized mainly by CYP 2B6 to metabolites 2-ethyl-5-methyl-3,3-diphenylpyrroline and 2-ethylidene-1,5-dimethyl-3,3-diphenylpyrrolidine, which are excreted in urine. Alteration of methadone levels can occur when combined with rifampin, phenothiazines, other narcotic analgesics, and CNS depressants.

Caution

Hepatic or renal impairment, hypothyroidism, Addison's disease, prostatic hypertrophy, urethral strictures, asthma, cor pulmonale, head injury. Not advised for use in pregnancy, during lactation, and in patients younger than 18 years of age.

BUPRENORPHINE

Chemical Group
Thebaine derivative

Trade Name
Buprenex (Reckitt-Benkiser)

Forms Available
Injections of 1 mL (0.3 mg buprenorphine)

Pharmacokinetics
Half-life is 1.2 to 7.2 hours (mean ~ 2.2 hours); peak effect in 1 hour; effect lasts for 6 hours.

Dispensing
Q.i.d. dosing as needed

Range of Dosing
Adults: 1 mL (0.3 mg buprenorphine) IM or slow IV injection every 6 hours as needed. Same 1-mL dose may be given 30 to 60 minutes after initial dose, if needed. In severe pain, 2 mL (0.6 mg buprenorphine) IM injection in a single dose may be given, providing stable patient response.

Children: 2 to 12 years: 2 to 6 μg per kg of body weight every 4 to 6 hours as needed. Not used in children younger than 2 years and never give repeat dose as in adults.

Elderly: start on lower dose of 0.5 mL (1.5 mg buprenorphine)

FDA Approval
Relief of severe to moderate pain, treatment of opioid withdrawal

Possible Mechanism of Action
Acts on mu opiate receptors in the CNS as a partial agonist. High affinity and slow dissociation from receptors prevents exogenous opioids (e.g., heroin, morphine) from exerting strong agonist effects.

Possible Advantages
- Safe in patients younger than 18 years
- No dependence
- Does not produce euphoria
- Diminishes cravings

Side Effects

- Sedation
- Nausea and vomiting
- Dizziness/vertigo
- Sweating
- Respiratory depression
- Hypotension
- Miosis
- Headache

Metabolism and Drug Interactions

Metabolized by the hepatic CYP 3A4 isozyme and excreted in urine. CYP 3A4 inhibitors (e.g., erythromycin, ketoconazole, protease inhibitors) can elevate buprenorphine levels. CYP 3A4 inducers (e.g., rifampin, carbamazepine, phenytoin) can decrease buprenorphine levels. CNS depressants, MAOI, and other opioid narcotics can cause exaggerated response when coadministration with buprenorphine

Caution

Severe hepatic, renal, or pulmonary impairment; Addison's disease; prostatic hypertrophy; urethral strictures; hypothyroidism; CNS depression; acute alcoholism

DISULFIRAM

Chemical Group
bis(diethylthiocarbamoyl) disulfide

Trade Name
Antabuse (Sidmak)

Forms Available
Tablets: 250 and 500 mg

Pharmacokinetics
Half-life is approximately 10 hours, but enzyme inhibiting effect can last longer (i.e., up to 14 days after discontinuation). Peak plasma level in 4 hours; peak enzyme inhibiting effect reached after 3 daily doses.

Dispensing
Q.i.d. dosing

Range of Dosing
Adults: initial dosing is a maximum of 500 mg daily, given in a single dose for 1 to 2 weeks. To minimize sedative effect, dose may be decreased. Never administer in acute alcohol intoxication. Average maintenance dose is 250 mg daily; range is 125 to 500 mg.
Children: not used.
Elderly: start at low end of dosing range; continue therapy until sustained self-control has been established.

FDA Approval
Alcohol dependence

Possible Mechanism of Action
Aversive clinical reaction that occurs with consumption of alcohol, due to the accumulation of acetaldehyde, makes disulfiram a deterrent to alcohol use. Use only in motivated and compliant patients as an adjunct to other supportive and psychotherapeutic interventions.

Possible Advantages
Only preparation available for alcohol abuse

Side Effects
- Polyneuritis, peripheral neuropathy, optic neuritis
- Psychosis (including manic episodes) with higher doses or due to combined toxicity with metronidazole or isoniazid

- In first 2 weeks of therapy: fatigue, transient sedation, headache, acneform eruption, allergic dermatitis, garlic or metallic aftertaste
- Hepatitis and hepatic necrosis

Metabolism and Drug Interactions

Metabolized in the liver to active metabolite diethylthiocarbaminic acid methyl ester. Excreted in urine and expired as carbon disulfide.

- Disulfiram-alcohol reaction: Inhibition of enzyme aldehyde dehydrogenase by disulfiram causes accumulation of acetaldehyde in body, following ingestion of alcohol. Within 10 minutes, the high level of acetaldehyde causes symptoms such as facial flushing, headaches, sweating, nausea, vomiting, chest pain, blurred vision, dizziness, and confusion. In severe reactions: respiratory depression, arrhythmias, shock, seizures, or death may occur. Intensity of reaction depends on amount of alcohol and disulfiram taken. Reaction lasts as long as alcohol is present in blood; may last up to several hours.
- Disulfiram decreases metabolism and raises blood levels of metronidazole, isoniazid, phenytoin, diazepam, and oral anticoagulants. Adjust doses accordingly.

Caution

Diabetes mellitus, hypothyroidism, epilepsy, cerebral damage, nephritis, hepatic cirrhosis

Contraindications

- Acute alcohol intoxication
- Myocardial disease; coronary occlusion
- Psychosis
- Rubber contact dermatitis (hypersensitivity to thiuram derivatives)
- Nursing mothers
- Alcohol-containing preparations, such as cough syrups, vinegar, aftershave lotions, tonics

Tests

Baseline and follow-up liver function tests, complete blood count, serum chemistries

Cholinesterase Inhibitors and Related Drugs for the Elderly

DONEPEZIL

Chemical Group
Piperidine derivative

Trade Name
Aricept (Pfizer)

Forms Available
Tablets of 5 and 10 mg

Pharmacokinetics
Half-life is 70 hours; peak plasma level in 3 to 4 hours. Steady state reached in 15 days

Dispensing
QD dosing

Range of Dosing
Initial dose is 5 mg per day for 1 to 4 weeks; then increase to 10 mg per day if drug is tolerated. Range is 5 to 10 mg. Increased incidence of adverse effects with 10 mg dosing as compared with 5 mg.

FDA Approval
Mild to moderate dementia of Alzheimer's type

Possible Mechanism of Action
Reversible acetlycholinesterase inhibitor

Possible Advantages
- Once per day dosing
- Improved cognitive function on the Alzheimer's Disease Assessment Scale (ADAS-cog) for as long as functioning cholinergic neurons remain intact; no alteration in actual disease process
- Fewer side effects and better tolerated than other cholinesterase inhibitors (e.g., rivastigmine, galantamine)
- Possible benefit in treatment of Down's syndrome

Side Effects

These are due to cholinergic effects and ususally resolve spontaneously.

- Nausea
- Diarrhea
- Insomnia
- Fatigue
- Vomiting
- Muscle cramps
- Anorexia
- Bradycardia

Metabolism and Drug Interactions

Metabolized in the liver by CYP 3A3/4 and CYP 2D6. It is primarily excreted in the urine. Drugs that inhibit the CYP 3A4 and CYP 2D6 enzymes (e.g., ketoconazole and quinidine) can inhibit metabolism of donepezil and increase levels. Inducers of these enzymes (e.g., phenytoin, carbamazepine, dexamethasone, rifampin, phenobarbital) can increase metabolism of donepezil and lower the plasma levels.

Caution

Coadministration with other cholinergic agonists can potentiate vagal effects such as bradycardia, gastric acid secretion, and bladder outflow obstruction. Use in pregnancy is done with caution due to possible teratogenic effect.

Tests

Heart rate monitoring before treatment. Close observation in patients with cardiac conduction delays or who are on beta-blockers recommended.

RIVASTIGMINE

Chemical Group
Carbamate derivative

Trade Name
Exelon (Novartis)

Forms Available
Capsules: 1.5, 3, 4.5, and 6 mg

Pharmacokinetics
Half-life is 1.5 hours; peak plasma level reached in 1 hour. Doubling the dose from 6 to 12 mg may cause three-fold rise in blood levels due to nonlinear elimination kinetics at higher dosing range. Clearance may decrease by more than 60% in patients with hepatic or renal impairment.

Dispensing
B.i.d. dosing with meals in morning and evening

Range of Dosing
Initially, 1.5 mg twice daily is given. May increase dose by 1.5 mg every 2 weeks provided patient is tolerant of adverse effects. Range is 6 to 12 mg per day.

FDA Approval
Mild to moderate dementia of Alzheimer's type

Possible Mechanism of Action
Reversible selective cholinesterase inhibitor

Possible Advantages
- Limits cognitive decline in patients with moderate disease
- More efficient than galantamine and donepezil in treating advanced stages of dementia due to nonselective inhibition of both acetylcholinesterase and butyryl-cholinesterase activity; butryrylcholinesterase activity is more predominant in advanced stages of dementia
- Effective in treating Lewy body dementia

Side Effects
Least tolerated of the cholinesterase inhibitors. Excessive central nervous selectivity causes increased amount of nausea and vomiting. Side effects are due to cholinergic

activity, including:

- Nausea and vomiting
- Diarrhea
- Anorexia
- Dizziness
- Headache
- Bradycardia
- Abdominal pain
- Fatigue

Metabolism and Drug Interactions

Metabolized by cholinesterase-mediated hydrolysis at site of target enzyme and excreted in urine. For this reason, drugs that are metabolized by the P450 isoenzymes do not interact with rivastigmine.

Caution

Due to cholinomimetic action, use with caution in cardiac conduction disorders, drugs that cause bradycardia, patients prone to ulcer disease or GI bleeding, and asthmatics. Not recommended in pregnancy due to possible teratogenic effect. Contraindicated in severe renal or hepatic impairment.

Tests

Heart rate monitoring before treatment. Close observation recommended in patients with cardiac conduction delays or who are on beta-blockers.

GALANTAMINE

Chemical Group

(4aS,6R,8aS)-4a,5,9,10,11,12-hexahydro-3-methoxy-11-methyl-6 H–bezofuro [3a, 3, 2ef] [2] benzazepin–6–ol hydrobromide

Trade Name

Reminyl (Janssen)

Forms Available

Tablets: 4, 8, and 12 mg; oral solution (4 mg per mL) in 100-mL bottle.

Pharmacokinetics

Half-life of 7 hours; peak plasma level reached in 1 hour. Oral bioavailability is 90% for both oral solution and tablet forms.

Dispensing

B.i.d. or t.i.d. dosing; taken with meals

Range of Dosing

Initially 4 mg twice per day; if well tolerated, increase dose to 8 mg twice per day after 4 weeks. Further dose increase after 4 additional weeks to 12 mg twice per day (or 8 mg three times daily), if needed. Range is 8 to 24 mg per day. In patients with moderate hepatic or renal impairment, dose should not exceed 16 mg per day.

FDA Approval

Mild to moderate dementia of Alzheimer's type

Possible Mechanism of Action

Reversible, competitive acetylcholinesterase inhibitor

Possible Advantages

- Mini-Mental State Examination score improvements greatest compared with other cholinesterase inhibitors
- Potential role in treatment of vascular dementia

Side Effects

These are due to cholinergic effects and usually resolve in 5 to 7 days:

- Nausea
- Vomiting
- Diarrhea
- Anorexia and weight loss

- Headache
- Bradycardia
- Fatigue

Metabolism and Drug Interaction

Metabolized in the liver by isoenzymes CYP 2D6 and CYP 3A4; excreted in urine. Concentrations increase with coadministration of drugs that inhibit these enzymes, such as paroxetine and ketoconazole. Severe renal impairment reduces the clearance of galantamine up to 66%.

Caution

Due to cholinomimetic action, use with caution in cardiac conduction disorders, drugs that cause bradycardia, patients prone to ulcer disease or GI bleeding, and asthmatics. Not recommended in pregnancy due to possible teratogenic effect. Contraindicated in severe renal or hepatic impairment.

Tests

Heart rate monitoring before treatment. Close observation recommended in patients with cardiac conduction delays or who are on beta-blockers.

MEMANTINE

Chemical Group
1-Amino-3,5-dimethyladamantane hydrochloride

Trade Name
Namenda (Forest)

Forms Available
Tablets: 5 and 10 mg; titration paks include 28 × 5 mg and 21 × 10 mg tablets.

Pharmacokinetics
Half-life of 60 to 80 hours; peak levels reached in 3 to 7 hours. Clearance is reduced with alkaline urine.

Dispensing
Once daily to start, then b.i.d. dosing

Range of Dosing
Initially, 5 mg once per day. Dose is increased by 5-mg increments in at least 1-week intervals to 10 mg per day (5 mg b.i.d.), 15 mg per day (5 and 10 mg as separate doses), and finally 20 mg per day (10 mg b.i.d.). Twenty mg per day is target dose. Dose should be lowered in moderate renal impairment. Use in severe renal impairment is not recommended.

FDA Approval
Moderate to severe dementia of Alzheimer's type

Possible Mechanism of Action
N-methyl-D-aspartate receptor antagonist. Provides neuroprotection by blocking glutamate excitotoxicity in brain, preventing calcium build-up.

Possible Advantages
• May be used in combination with cholinesterase inhibitors due to different mechanism of action
• Improves activities of daily living, social behavior, and lack of drive, as well as cognitive function
• Possible benefit in treatment of chronic pain, drug cravings, dementia in AIDS, multiple sclerosis, and glaucoma is being researched

Side Effects
• Frequent: confusion, dizziness, headache, fatigue, hallucination

• Infrequent: anxiety, hypertonus, vomiting, bladder infection, increased sex drive

Metabolism and Drug Interactions

Majority (57% to 82%) of memantine is not metabolized and is excreted unchanged in the urine. The remaining portion is metabolized to inactive metabolites in the liver. Metabolism is not done through the P450 enzyme system. Levels may rise with coadministration of drugs that alkalinize urine (e.g., carbonic anhydrase inhibitors, sodium bicarbonate). Drug interactions may also occur with drugs that undergo elimination by the same renal mechanism (e.g., hydrochlorothiazide, triamterene, cimetidine, ranitidine, guanidine).

Contraindications

Severe renal or hepatic impairment, pregnancy, hypersensitivity to memantine

Caution

Conditions with raised urinary pH

Miscellaneous Medications

PROPRANOLOL

Chemical Group
1-(Isopropylamino)-3-(1-naphthyloxy)-2-propanol

Trade Name
Inderal (Wyeth-Ayerst)

Forms Available
Tablets: 10, 20, 40, 60, 80, and 90 mg; long-acting tablets: 60, 80, 120, and 160 mg; injectable: 1 mg per mL.

Pharmacokinetics
Half-life approximately 4 hours; peak effect in 1 to 1.5 hours

Dispensing
B.i.d. or t.i.d. dosing

Range of Dosing
Adults: 10–120 mg per day
Children: Usually 2 to 8 mg per kg per day, up to three times per day.
Elderly: no specific dose range has been established for psychotropic use.

FDA Approval
- Management of hypertension
- Long-term treatment of angina pectoris
- Supraventricular arrythmias: paroxsysmal atrial tachycardia, Wolff-Parkinson-White syndrome, persistent sinus tachycardia, thyrotoxic arrythmias, persistent atrial extrasystoles, atrial flutter and fibrillation
- Ventricular tachycardia that is not caused by catecholamines or digitalis

Possible Mechanism of Action
Nonselective, beta-adrenergic receptor blocker agent

Possible Advantages
- Drug of choice for akathisia
- Commonly used in psychiatry for reducing arousal and agitation: Tourette's, ADHD, aggression, self-abuse

Side Effects

- CV: hypotension, bradycardia
- CNS: mental depression, light-headedness, amnesia, emotional liability, confusion, hallucinations, dizziness, fatigue, insomnia, hypersomnolence, psychosis, cognitive dysfunction
- Skin: rash, alopecia, exfoliative dermatitis, hyperkeratosis
- Endocrine system: hypoglycemia or hyperglycemia, lipid abnormalities, hyperkalemia
- GIT: diarrhea, nausea, vomiting, stomach discomfort, constipation, anorexia
- Hematology: agranulocytosis, thrombocytopenia
- Respiratory system: wheezing, bronchospasam, pulmonary edema
- Ocular: mydriasis, decreased production of tears, hyperemia of conjunctiva, decreased visual acuity

Metabolism and Drug Interactions

Extensive first-pass metabolism. Metabolized in liver by CYP 12A, 2C18, and 2D6 into active and inactive compounds. Blunted effect with nonspecific beta-agonists. Concurrent use with alpha-blocker increases risk of orthostasis.

Caution

Diabetes, glaucoma, thyrotoxicosis

Contraindications

Bronchial asthma, congestive heart failure, cardiogenic shock, and sinus bradycardia, and greater than first-degree heart block.

DESMOPRESSIN

Chemical Group
A synthetic analogue of natural antidiuretic hormone (D-arginine vasopressin monoacetate trihydrate)

Trade Name
DDAVP (Rhone-Poulenc Rorer)

Forms Available
Tablets: 0.1 and 0.2 mg; nasal spray: 100 mcg per mL nasal.

Pharmacokinetics
Half-life is 75 minutes; onset of action in 1 hour with peak effect seen in 1 to 5 hours; duration of action is 5 to 21 hours

Dispensing
QHS dosing

Range of Dosing
Children age 6 years or older for nocturnal enuresis: initial dosage of 0.2 mg (0.2 mL) at bedtime. Half dose is given in each nostril. Range is 0.1 to 0.4 mg.
Elderly: no information available.

FDA Approval
Enuresis

Possible Mechanism of Action
Like the naturally occurring hormone, DDAVP binds to Vasopressin (V2) receptor sites in the collecting ducts of the kidneys. Thus, increases the cellular permeability of the collecting duct to H_2O. By enhancing reabsorption, DDAVP achieves an antidiuretic effect, decreasing urine volume and increasing urine concentration (osmolality).

Possible Advantages
DDAVP is used for enuresis.

Side Effects
1% to 10%: facial flushing, headache, dizziness, nausea, abdominal cramps, nasal congestion
Less than 1%: hyponatremia, elevated blood pressure, water intoxication

Metabolism and Drug Interactions

Metabolism is unknown. Demeclocycline and lithium may decrease ADH effect. Chlorpropamide and fludrocortisone may increase ADH effect.

Tests

Periodic sodium levels

Medication Clinic Progress Note Format

Vital Signs
BP, pulse, weight, and height

Target Symptoms (index/present)

Intervention-Effect (present/future-reasoning)
- Biological:
  - Medication
  - Effect
  - Side effects
  - Patient education (what, what for, when, how much)
- Psychological
- Social
- School/work
- Liaison with other agencies involved

Risk of Tardive Dyskinesia
Explained where relevant—Yes/NA

B Lithium Laboratory Monitor

Patient's name _____ — Height _____

Date	Ratings		Form of lithium and dose	No. of hours since last dose	Test (frequency)								
	Depression 0-6	Mania 0-6			Serum lithium (q 2 mo + prn)	Serum creatinine (q 6 mo)	Urine-specific gravity (q 6 mo)	24-Hr urine volume (q 6 mo)	T₄RIA (q 1 yr)	T₃RU (q 1 yr)	TSH (q 1 yr)	Weight (q 1 yr)

Frequency of monitoring depends on many factors and may be done more or less often. Stable patients are usually monitored less often.

C Abnormal Involuntary Movement Scale—Modified (AIMS-M3D)

Patient's name _____ Date _____ Medications _____

Code: 0 = none; 1 = minimal, maybe extreme normal; 2 = mild; 3 = moderate; 4 = severe (ratings for maximum movement during rating period);
A = movement present only during activation; NR = not ratable.

Body Region	Not Ratable	Abnormal (yes/no)?	Choreo-athetosis	Dystonia	Movement Type (Circle if appropriate)	Tic*	Mannerism/ stereotypy	Tremor	Other (specify)
			Tardive Dyskinesia–Like Movements			Non-Tardive Dyskinesia–Like Movements			
1. Muscles of facial expression	NR	Y/N	0 1 2 3 4 A	0 1 2 3 4	Movements of forehead, eyebrows, or periorbital area; include frowning, blinking**	0 1 2 3 4	0 1 2 3 4	0 1 2 3 4	0 1 2 3 4
2. Lips and perioral region	NR	Y/N	0 1 2 3 4 A	0 1 2 3 4	Puckering, pouting, smacking, cheeks puff out	0 1 2 3 4	0 1 2 3 4	0 1 2 3 4	0 1 2 3 4
3. Jaw	NR	Y/N	0 1 2 3 4 A	0 1 2 3 4	Biting, clenching, chewing, mouth opening	0 1 2 3 4	0 1 2 3 4	0 1 2 3 4	0 1 2 3 4
4. Tongue	NR	Y/N	0 1 2 3 4 A	0 1 2 3 4	Movements only in and out of mouth	0 1 2 3 4	0 1 2 3 4	0 1 2 3 4	0 1 2 3 4
5. Upper extremities	NR	Y/N	R. 0 1 2 3 4 A L. 0 1 2 3 4 A	0 1 2 3 4 0 1 2 3 4	Arm, wrist, hand, fingers Arm, wrist, hand, fingers	0 1 2 3 4 0 1 2 3 4	0 1 2 3 4 0 1 2 3 4	0 1 2 3 4 0 1 2 3 4	0 1 2 3 4 0 1 2 3 4

(Continued)

C Abnormal Involuntary Movement Scale—Modified (AIMS-M3D) (Continued)

		Tardive Dyskinesia–Like Movements				Non-Tardive Dyskinesia–Like Movements			
Body Region	Not Ratable	Abnormal (yes/no)?	Choreo-athetosis	Dystonia	Movement Type (Circle if appropriate)	Tic*	Mannerism/ stereotypy	Tremor	Other (specify)
6. Lower extremities	NR	Y/N R. L.	0 1 2 3 4 A 0 1 2 3 4 A	0 1 2 3 4 0 1 2 3 4	Legs, knees, ankles, toes, lateral knee movement, foot tapping, heel dropping, foot squirming, inversion and eversion of foot	0 1 2 3 4 0 1 2 3 4	0 1 2 3 4 0 1 2 3 4	0 1 2 3 4 0 1 2 3 4	0 1 2 3 4 0 1 2 3 4
7. Trunk	NR	Y/N	0 1 2 3 4 A	0 1 2 3 4	Neck, shoulders, hips, rocking, twisting, pelvic gyrations, diaphragm	0 1 2 3 4	0 1 2 3 4	0 1 2 3 4	0 1 2 3 4

General Tardive Dyskinesia–Like Rating Items (1–7) 0 1 2 3 4	*Tics may occasionally be part of tardive dyskinesia. **Increased blinking may be part of a psychotic illness.	8. Bradykinesia (Y/N)? R. 0 1 2 3 4 L. 0 1 2 3 4	9. Rigidity (Y/N)? R. 0 1 2 3 4 L. 0 1 2 3 4	10. Loss of facial expression 0 1 2 3 4	11. Abnormal gait and posture 0 1 2 3 4	12. Akathisia 0 1 2 3 4
Patient awareness 0 1 2 3 4 Incapacitation 0 1 2 3 4	Problems with teeth/dentures (Y/N)? If "yes," what kind?	Date:				
TOTAL Tardive Dyskinesia–Like Score (1–7) (use average of both sides for items 5 and 6) Choreoathetosis _____ Dystonia _____	Previous Total AIMS Scores:					

D Pediatric Side Effects Checklist (P-SEC)

This Checklist is to be completed by parent, child or patient. This will help to identify the adverse effects of the medications. Please read through the list and check (✓) in the appropriate box.

Patient Name:		Id:		Date:	

PROBLEMS	NONE	MILD/ SOMETIMES BUT TOLERABLE	MODERATE/ INTERFERES SOMEWHAT	SEVERE/ INTERFERES A LOT
Gastrointestinal system				
Discomfort in the stomach				
Constipation				
Diarrhea				
Increased appetite				
Decreased appetite				
Nausea/Vomiting				
Central Nervous system				
Muscle trembling/Shaking				
Sleepiness				
Difficulty falling asleep				
Muscle stiffness				
Stiff jaw				

(Continued)

D Pediatric Side Effects Checklist (P-SEC) (Continued)

Problems	None	Mild/ Sometimes but Tolerable	Moderate/ Interferes Somewhat	Severe/ Interferes a Lot
Problem concentrating				
Problems with memory				
Restlessness/wanting to pace				
Irritable/Agitated				
Problems with speech				
Dizziness/Lightheadedness				
Headache				
Seizures				
Nightmares/Vivid dreams				
Blurring of vision				
Excessive drooling				
Increased sweating				
Dry mouth/eyes				
Skin				
Rash				
Acne				
Hair loss				

Cardiovascular system			
Palpitations			
Blackouts/loss of consciousness			
Chest pain			
Endocrine system			
Feeling cold /hot			
Weight gain			
Weight loss			
Fatigue/Tiredness			
Breast cyst			
Changes in menstrual periods			
Mood /Behavior Changes			
Depression/feeling sad			
Excitable			
Feeling anxious			
Aggressive			
Panic attacks			
Renal system			
Increased urination			
Bed wetting			
Frothy urine/red colored urine			
Sexual concerns/problems			

(Continued)

D Pediatric Side Effects Checklist (P-SEC) (*Continued*)

Please indicate your current medications here

MEDICATION	Dose

This checklist (P-SEC) accounts for most of the possible side effects seen with medications utilized in psychopharmacotherapy.
For comments e-mail to: mpavuluri@psych.uic.edu

Abbreviations

A
A, Adrenergic
ADAS, Alzheimer's disease assessment scale
ADHD, Attention-deficit hyperactivity disorder
ANS, Autonomic nervous system

B
BUN, Blood urea nitrogen
BZD, Benzodiazepine

C
cAMP, Cyclic adenosine monophosphate
CBC, Complete blood cell count
CBZ, Carbamazepine
CD, Controlled delivery
CMP, Complete metabolic profile
CNS, Central nervous system
CR, Controlled release
CVS, Cardiovascular system
CYP, Cytochrome P

D
D, Dopamine
DA, Dopamine and adrenergic
DARI, Dopamine and adrenergic reuptake inhibitor
DKA, Diabetic ketoacidosis
DRI, Dopamine reuptake inhibitor

E
ECG, Electrocardiogram
ER, Extended release
ESR, Erythrocyte sedimentation rate

F
FDA, Food and Drug Administration
FGA, First-generation antipsychotics

G
GABA, gamma-aminobutyric acid
GAD, General anxiety disorder
GFR, Glomerular filtration rate
GGT, Gamma glutamyl transferase
GI, Gastrointestinal
GIT, Gastrointestinal tract

H
HCA, Heterocyclic
HCG, Human chorionic gonadotropin
HIV, Human immunodeficiency virus

I
IR, Immediate release

L
LFT, Liver function test

M
MAOI, Monoamine oxidase inhibitor
MHD, 10-Monohydroxy metabolite
MI, Myocardial infarction

N
NaSSA, Noradrenergic and specific serotonergic antagonist
NE, Norepinephrine
NRI, Norepinephrine reuptake inhibitor
NSAID, Nonsteroidal antiinflammatory drug

O
OCD, Obsessive-compulsive disorder

P
PCOS, Polycystic ovarian syndrome
PIP, Phosphoinositol phosphate
PKC, Protein kinase C
PMDD, Premenstrual dysphoric disorder
PMNL, Polymorphonuclear leukocytes
PTSD, Posttraumatic stress disorder

R
RFT, Renal function test

S
SARI, Serotonin-adrenergic reuptake inhibitor
S-CT, S-enantiomer of citalopram
SGPT, Serum glutamate pyruvate transferase
SIADH, Syndrome of inappropriate antidiuretic hormone
SNRI, Serotonin and norepinephrine reuptake inhibitor
SR, Sustained release
SRI, Serotonin reuptake inhibitor
SSRI, Selective serotonin reuptake inhibitor

T
T_3, Thyroxine
T_4, Thyronine
TFT, Thyroid function test
TSH, Thyroid-stimulating hormone

W
WBC, White blood (cell) count

X
XR, Extended release

Newly-released Drug: Symbyax

OLANZAPINE PLUS FLUOXETINE

Chemical Group
2-methyl-4-(4-methyl-1-piperazinyl)-10H-thieno[2,3-b][1, 5]benzodiazepine.

Trade Name
Symbyax (Eli lilly)

Forms Available
Capsules of olanzapine and fluoxetine hydrochloride (OFC) in four dosage options:
Olanzapine 6 mg plus Fluoxetine 25 mg
Olanzapine 6 mg plus Fluoxetine 50 mg
Olanzapine 12 mg plus Fluoxetine 25 mg
Olanzapine 12 mg plus Fluoxetine 50 mg

Dispensing
Usually taken once a day in the evening. May be taken with or without food.

Range of Dosing
Adults: Should be administered once daily in the evening, generally beginning with the 6-mg/25-mg capsule. While food has no appreciable effect on the absorption of olanzapine and fluoxetine given individually, the effect of food on its absorption has not been studied. Dosage adjustments, if indicated, can be made according to efficacy and tolerability. Antidepressant efficacy was demonstrated in a dose range of olanzapine 6 to 12 mg and fluoxetine 25 to 50 mg
Children: No information available
Elderly: No information available

FDA Approval
Bipolar depression

Possible Mechanisms of Action
It is the same as those of olanzapine and fluoxetine.
Mechanism of action is unknown but it has been proposed that the monoaminergic neural systems (serotonin, dopamine and norepinephrine) are responsible for enhanced antidepressant effect.

Possible Advantages

Using a single drug as mood stabilizer, offering the additional advantage of actively addressing depressive symptoms in bipolar disorder

Side Effects

Most common side effects are somnolence (22%), weight gain (21%), increased appetite (16%) and asthenia (15%)

Drug Interactions

Should not be used with in 14 days of discontinuing MAOI. At least 5 weeks are allowed after stopping this agent before using MAOI.

Reference

Janicak PG, Davis JM, Perskorn SH, et al. *Principles and practice of psychopharmacotherapy,* 3rd ed. Philadelphia: Lippincott Williams & Wilkins, 2001.

Subject Index

Note: Boldface numbers indicate tables or figures.